Visual Guide for Clinicians
BLOOD PRESSURE MANAGEMENT AND STROKE PREVENTION

Visual Guide for Clinicians

BLOOD PRESSURE MANAGEMENT AND STROKE PREVENTION

Isaac E Silverman, MD
Vascular Neurology
Co-Medical Director
The Stroke Center at Hartford Hospital
Hartford, Connecticut
USA

Marilyn M Rymer, MD
Mid-America Brain and Stroke Institute
Saint Luke's Hospital
UKMC School of Medicine
Kansas City, Missouri
USA

Luis M Ruilope, MD, PhD, FESC
Chair, ESC Working Group on Cardiovascular
Pharmacology and Drug Therapy
Hypertension Unit
Hospital 12 de Octubre
Madrid
Spain

CLINICAL PUBLISHING

OXFORD

Clinical Publishing
an imprint of Atlas Medical Publishing Ltd
Oxford Centre for Innovation
Mill Street, Oxford OX2 0JX, UK

Tel: +44 1865 811116
Fax: +44 1865 251550
Email: info@clinicalpublishing.co.uk
Web: www.clinicalpublishing.co.uk

ISBN   978 1 84692 103 2
eISBN   978 1 84692 646 4

**The publisher makes no representation, express or implied, that the dosages
in this book are correct. Readers must therefore always check the product
information and clinical procedures with the most up-to-date published product
information and data sheets provided by the manufacturers and the most recent
codes of conduct and safety regulations. The authors and the publisher do not
accept any liability for any errors in the text or for the misuse or misapplication
of material in this work.**

Project manager: Gavin Smith, GPS Publishing Solutions, Herts, UK
Illustrations by Graeme Chambers, BA(Hons)
Typeset by Phoenix Photosetting, Chatham, Kent, UK
Printed by Marston Book Services Ltd, Abingdon, Oxon, UK

Contents

Acknowledgements

We are indebted to many physicians and other professional colleagues for their comments on the evolving manuscript as well as their contributions to the images included in the book. Our sincere thanks to Robert Schmidt, MD, PhD, Professor of Pathology and Immunology at Washington University School of Medicine. Many of the beautiful pathology photos are his. We also had excellent assistance from Dean Uphoff, MD of the Pathology Department at Hartford Hospital and Louis R. Caplan, MD at the Beth Israel-Deaconess Medical Center in Boston.

The strength of this project is based on the cases and neurovascular pathology that are evaluated on a weekly basis at the multidisciplinary Neurovascular Clinic of Hartford Hospital. Colleagues in this clinic are Donna Avanecean, Neurovascular APRN; Drs Kureshi and Spiegel; and in Vascular Neurology, Nora S. Lee, MD and Louise D. McCullough, MD, PhD.

The other chief source of case studies for this textbook is the inpatient service of the Stroke Center at Hartford Hospital. Core members not mentioned above from our stroke team are Dawn Beland, RN; Joao A. Gomes, MD; Stephen K. Ohki, MD; Lincoln Abbott, MD; A. Jon Smally, MD; Michele Landes, RN; and our clinical trials coordinators, Martha Ahlquist, LPN, and Jennifer Blum.

A special thanks to Krzysztof Dzialo of the Radiology File Room, and Vladilen Bokotey, Radiology systems manager, both at Hartford Hospital. The input from these two individuals made feasible the digital manipulation of the many MRI, CT and angiographic studies that form the heart of this book.

We would also like to thank the following for their valuable assistance: L. Christy Turtzo, MD, PhD; Gary R. Spiegel, MD; Naveed Akhtar, MD; Ethan Foxman, MD; Inam U. Kureshi, MD; Paul Gaudio, MD; and Cynthia Taub, MD.

Abbreviations

ACA	anterior cerebral artery
ACCESS	Acute Candesartan Cilexetil Therapy in Stroke Survivors (clinical trial)
ACE	angiotensin-converting enzyme
AChA	anterior choroidal artery
ACoA	anterior communicating artery
ADH	anti-diuretic hormone
AICA	anterior inferior cerebellar artery
AIS	acute ischemic stroke
AMPA	α-amino-3-hydroxy-5-methyl-4-isoxazole propionic acid
AP	anteroposterior
ARB	angiotensin receptor blocker
AT_1	angiotensin II receptor type 1
BA	basilar artery
BI	Barthel Index
BP	blood pressure
BPLTTC	Blood Pressure Lowering Treatment Trialists' Collaboration
CADASIL	cerebral autosomal dominant arteriopathy with subcortical infarcts and leukoencephalopathy
CAPRIE	Clopidogrel vs Aspirin in Patients at Risk of Ischemic Events (clinical trial)
CCB	calcium channel blocker
CHARISMA	Clopidogrel for High Atherothrombotic Risk and Ischemic Stabilization, Management, and Avoidance (clinical trial)
CI	confidence interval
CNS	central nervous system
CSF	cerebrospinal fluid
CTA	computed tomography angiography
CT	computed tomography
DBP	diastolic blood pressure
DW-MRI	diffusion-weighted MRI sequence
ECA	external carotid artery
E-COST	Efficacy of Candesartan on Outcome in Saitama Trial
EMS	Emergency Medical Services
ESC	European Society of Cardiology
ESH	European Society of Hypertension
ESPRIT	European/Australasian Stroke Prevention in Reversible Ischaemia Trial (clinical trial)
ESPS-2	European Stroke Prevention Study 2 (clinical trial)
ETA	type A endothelin receptor
FDA	Food and Drug Administration
FLAIR MRI	fluid-attenuated inversion recovery MRI sequence
FMD	fibromuscular dysplasia
GCA	giant cell arteritis
GE MRI	gradient echo MRI sequence
GOS	Glasgow Outcome Scale
HD	hospital day
IA	intra-arterial
ICA	internal carotid artery
ICH	intracerebral hemorrhage
ICU	intensive care unit
IDR	incidence density ratio
INR	international normalized ratio
IP_3	inositol trisphosphate
IV	intravenous
LDL	low-density lipoprotein
LIFE	Losartan Intervention for Endpoint reduction (clinical trial)
LVH	left ventricular hypertrophy
MATCH	Management of Atherothrombosis with Clopidogrel in High-Risk Patients with Recent Transient Ischemic Attacks or Ischemic Stroke (clinical trial)
MCA	middle cerebral artery
MELAS	mitochondrial encephalopathy, lactic acidosis, and stroke-like episodes
MERCI	Mechanical Embolus Removal in Cerebral Ischemia (clinical trial)
MI	myocardial infarction
MOSES	Morbidity and Mortality After Stroke: Eprosartan Compared with Nitrendipine for Secondary Prevention
MRA	magnetic resonance angiography
MRI	magnetic resonance imaging
mRS	modified Rankin Scale
NAVIGATOR	Nateglinide and Valsartan in Impaired Glucose Tolerance Outcomes Research (clinical trial)
NIHSS	National Institutes of Health Stroke Scale

NINDS	National Institutes of Neurologic Disease and Stroke	PT/INR	prothrombin time (international normalized ratio)
NINDS rt-PA	NINDS Recombinant Tissue Plasminogen Activator (clinical trial)	RAAS	renin-angiotensin-aldosterone system
NMDA	N-methyl-D-aspartate	RAS	renin-angiotensin system
NO	nitric oxide	RCT	randomized controlled trial
ONTARGET	Ongoing Telmisartan Alone and in Combination with Ramipril Global Endpoint Trial	SAH	subarachnoid hemorrhage
		SBP	systolic blood pressure
		SCAST	Scandinavian Candesartan Acute Stroke Trial
OS	oculus sinister (left eye)	SCA	superior cerebellar artery
PAI	plasminogen activator inhibitor	SCOPE	Study on Cognition and Prognosis in the Elderly
PCA	posterior cerebral artery		
PCoA	posterior communicating artery	SILVHIA	Swedish Irbesartan Left Ventricular Hypertrophy Investigation versus Atenolol
PFO	patent foramen ovale		
PHQ-9	Patient Health Questionnaire (nine-item)	Syst-Eur	Systolic Hypertension in Europe (clinical trial)
PICA	posterior inferior cerebellar artery	TEE	transesophageal echocardiogram
PROACT-II	Prolyse in Acute Cerebral Thromboembolism II (clinical trial)	TIA	transient ischemic attack
		TOAST	Trial of ORG10172 in Acute Stroke Treatment (clinical trial)
PRoFESS	Prevention Regimen for Effectively Avoiding Second Strokes (clinical trial)	t-PA	tissue plasminogen activator
		VALUE	Valsartan Antihypertensive Long-term Use Evaluation (clinical trial)
PROGRESS	Perindopril Protection Against Recurrent Stroke Study	VA	vertebral artery

Chapter 1

Stroke Basics

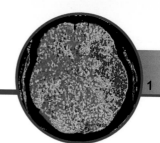

Introduction

Stroke is the second leading cause of death worldwide and the leading cause of adult disability in many countries. It is imperative that all physicians understand the basics of stroke diagnosis and treatment for three reasons:

- Stroke occurs as an acute event, and people will access the closest medical facility or physician's office for help. Primary care and emergency medicine physicians need to be able to rapidly diagnose and treat patients with acute stroke symptoms.
- Emerging treatments for stroke are time-dependent. The earlier the initiation of treatment, the better the outcome.
- Once a stroke has occurred, the risk of a second stroke increases. It is essential that clinicians identify and treat the stroke mechanism and risk factors and institute medications (e.g., antithrombotic and blood pressure-lowering agents) when appropriate in order to prevent recurrence.

The goal of this atlas is to provide clinicians and students with a foundation in the clinical presentation, neuroimaging, pathology, pathophysiology, and treatment of stroke syndromes and neurovascular disorders so that they can make an accurate diagnosis and initiate treatment and/or seek vascular neurology consultation when appropriate.

What is a stroke?

A stroke is caused by a disruption in the flow of blood to part of the brain either because of occlusion of a blood vessel in the case of acute ischemic stroke (AIS) or the rupture of a blood vessel causing bleeding in or around the brain: intracerebral hemorrhage (ICH) or subarachnoid hemorrhage (SAH), respectively (**1.1**). When stroke symptoms resolve and do not cause permanent brain damage, they are called a transient ischemic attack (TIA). Although the historical definition of a TIA is neurological symptoms lasting less than 24 hours, the duration of most TIAs is between 5 and 30 minutes, and can be considered a cerebral equivalent of cardiac angina.[1] Some healthcare professionals and patients refer to TIAs as 'mini-strokes,' but a TIA is actually a warning that a stroke may occur very soon.

Stroke epidemiology

Stroke incidence and mortality are increasing along with modernization and advancing longevity. Worldwide, 15 million people suffer a stroke each year. Five million of those die and 5 million are left permanently disabled.[2] It is estimated that by 2020, stroke mortality will have almost doubled as a result of an aging population and the future effects of current smoking patterns.[3]

Two-thirds of all stroke deaths and 60% of all strokes occur in low and middle income countries.[4] As infectious diseases and malnutrition decline in developing countries, stroke incidence rises due to decreased physical activity, increased tobacco use, and dietary changes. By 2040 there will be a billion adults aged 65 years or older at risk for stroke in low and middle income countries. In addition to the aging population, the major stroke risk factors worldwide are hypertension and tobacco use. In most countries, up to 30% of adults suffer from hypertension.[2] Men have a slightly higher incidence of stroke than women, but women have higher mortality rates. Black people have a higher stroke mortality rate than white people, and the mortality rate for Hispanic people falls between that of white and black people. There is a high incidence of hemorrhagic stroke in Asian people.[3]

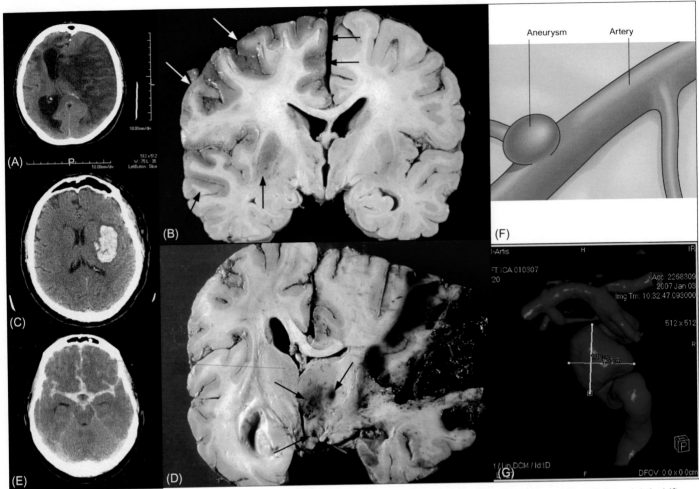

1.1 Major stroke subtypes. (A) Acute ischemic stroke. Hypodense infarct on head CT scan, with extensive midline (left-to-right) shift. (B) Subacute ischemic stroke. Gross pathology, at 3–4 days, in the territory of the internal carotid artery (ICA). Note edema and altered gray–white matter differentiation in the distribution of the MCA and ACA territories (arrows). (C) Primary intracerebral hemorrhage. A hyperdense lesion on CT scan located in the left putamen is a typical location for hypertensive hemorrhage due to small vessel disease. (D) Intracerebral hemorrhage. Gross pathology of a frontoparietal intracerebral hemorrhage resulting in subfalcine and uncal herniation; mass effect likely caused deep midline, punctate lesions, known as Duret hemorrhages (arrows). (E) Subarachnoid hemorrhage. CT scan reveals hyperdense blood diffusely filling the subarachnoid spaces around the Circle of Willis and the Sylvian fissures, bilaterally, and the interhemispheric fissure. (F) Intracranial aneurysm: an illustration. (G) Aneurysm of the carotid artery. A large aneurysm of the cavernous portion of the ICA is measured on a three-dimensional rendering of the conventional angiogram. The distal branches of the ICA, the MCA (extending laterally, to the left), and the ACA (extending medially) are also shown at the top of this image. The right side of the image is labeled 'R.' Pathology courtesy of Robert Schmidt MD, PhD.

Strokes occur at any age, but are more common in the elderly. Stroke risk doubles with every decade beyond 50 years of age, but 30% of strokes occur before the age of 65 in the USA.

Types of stroke

Ischemic stroke

Ischemic stroke, the most common type, is caused by an occlusion of an artery in the neck or in the brain, depriving a part of the brain of its nutrients, glucose and oxygen. The etiologies for AIS are diverse (**1.2**). The arterial occlusion is most often caused by a thrombus that has traveled to the brain (embolized) from a more proximal location in the body, such as the heart or from plaque in the wall of a proximal artery, such as the aorta or the internal carotid artery.[5] Less often, the etiology is a local thrombus developing immediately at the site of occlusion

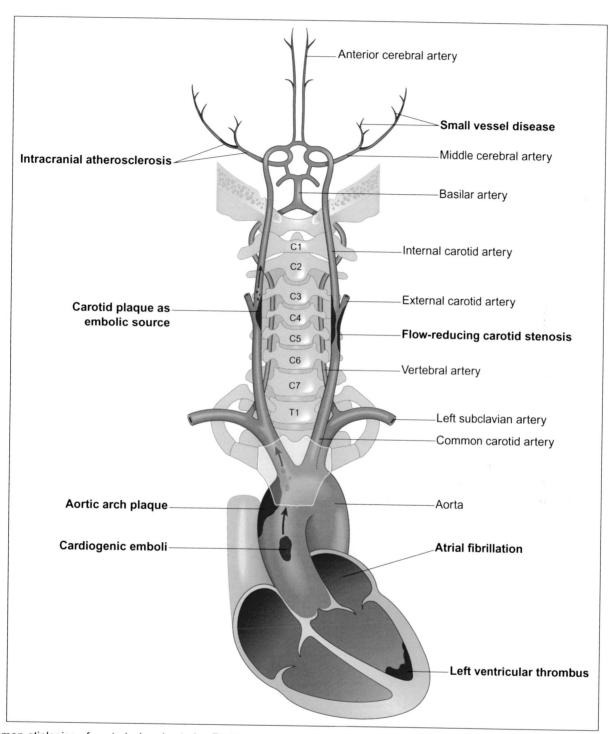

1.2 Common etiologies of acute ischemic stroke. Redrawn with permission from Albers *et al.*[5]

in large intracranial arteries (middle cerebral or basilar) or in small penetrating vessels, referred to as small vessel disease. Ischemic strokes account for 80–85% of strokes in most parts of the world, except for Asia, where ICH is more common.

Hemorrhagic stroke

ICH is caused by the rupture of a blood vessel, with bleeding directly into brain parenchyma, the ventricles, and/or spaces around the brain (**1.1C,D**). The rupture can occur because of acquired disease of the small penetrating arteries most commonly related to long-standing hypertension (small vessel disease), degenerative disease of superficial arteries (amyloid angiopathy), or from structural abnormalities of larger intracranial arteries, such as arteriovenous malformations. SAH occurs when an intracranial aneurysm ruptures and blood invades the spaces around the brain (**1.1E–G**). Aneurysms are balloon-shaped outpouchings of an artery where the vessel's wall has weakened.

Stroke symptoms

The reference list at the end of this chapter lists a number of textbooks that provide more detail on clinical stroke syndromes.[6–8] The hallmark of stroke is *sudden onset of neurologic deficit*. Individual stroke symptoms depend entirely on what anatomical area of the central nervous system (brain, spinal cord, or eye) is damaged. Usually, stroke presents as a syndrome, a collection of symptoms that help the examiner localize the region of the central nervous system that is acutely injured.

1 *Headache.* Sudden severe headache is often associated with ICH and SAH, but is uncommon in ischemic stroke. An exception is ischemic stroke caused by carotid or vertebral artery dissection in which headache, facial, or neck pain are typical.[9,10]
2 *Weakness.* A sudden decrease in motor strength is the most common symptom of stroke.[11] The National Institutes of Health Stroke Scale (NIHSS) grading for motor strength (0–4) is a good way to reliably document the degree of limb weakness (*Table 1.1*).[12] Several terms are frequently used to describe stroke-related weakness (*Table 1.2*).

The degree of weakness usually depends on where in the motor system the lesion occurs. Peripheral cortical lesions may produce only focal weakness (paresis), most commonly involving the face and/or arm, or even the hand or individual fingers in isolation (**1.3A,B**). More proximal, subcortical or brainstem lesions usually cause a more uniform weakness of the face, arm, and leg on one side of the body (hemiparesis) due to the tight collection of motor tracts in those locations. Upper motor neuron lesions of the motor cortex may result in downstream atrophy of the motor pathways in the ipsilateral cerebral peduncle, called Wallerian degeneration (**1.3C**).

Table 1.1 NIH Stroke Scale (NIHSS) Score (www.ninds.nih.gov/doctors/NIH_stroke_scale.pdf)

1 Level of consciousness is tested by clinical observation, response to two questions and ability to follow two commands. 5 points
2 Best gaze assesses eye movements. 2 points
3 Visual fields. 3 points
4 Facial movements. 3 points
5 Hemiparesis and hemiplegia in upper and lower extremities
6 Each limb is graded individually (4 points for each limb)
• 0—patient can extend the arm (10 seconds) and leg (5 seconds) in the air without drifting downward. This indicates no weakness
• 1—patient can extend the extremity but there is downward drift; the limb does not fall to the table
• 2—patient can extend the extremity but the limb drops to the table
• 3—patient cannot extend the extremity against gravity, but there is volitional movement
• 4—patient cannot move the limb volitionally

The term paresis describes NIHSS grades 1, 2 and 3; and plegia describes NIHSS grade 4.

7 Ataxia is assessed in each limb (2 points)
8 Sensation is assessed on both sides of the body (2 points)
9 Language (presence of aphasia) is tested (3 points)
10 Dysarthria (2 points)
11 Extinction (formerly 'neglect') (2 points)

Table 1.2 Weakness associated with stroke

• Monoparesis: weakness of one limb
• Hemiparesis: weakness of both limbs on one side of the body
• Monoplegia: paralysis of one limb
• Hemiplegia: paralysis of both limbs on one side of the body
• Paraparesis: weakness of both legs
• Paraplegia: paralysis of both legs

Note: Paraparesis or paraplegia can result from ischemic or hemorrhagic stroke of the spinal cord, and rarely, bilateral anterior cerebral artery territory infarction.

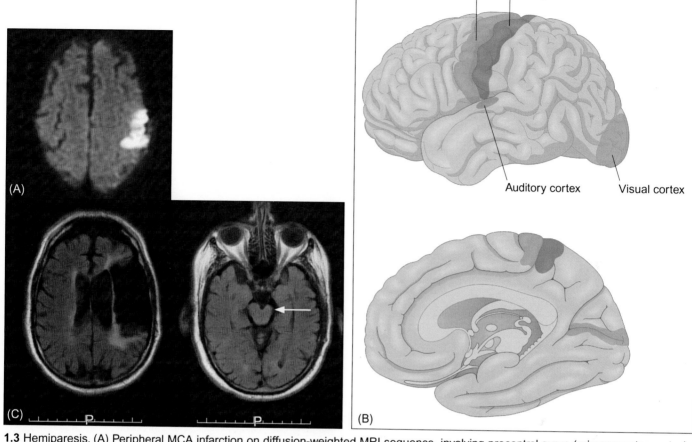

1.3 Hemiparesis. (A) Peripheral MCA infarction on diffusion-weighted MRI sequence, involving precentral gyrus (primary motor cortex). (B) Illustration of motor and sensory strips in the brain cortex. (C) Chronic left MCA-territory stroke, resulting in a wide region of encephalomalacia on the FLAIR MRI sequence (left). Atrophy of the ipsilateral cerebral peduncle (arrow), demonstrates associated Wallerian degeneration (right).

Most motor recovery from stroke occurs during the initial 1–3 months.[13] Incremental gains, however, can be made over the subsequent 9 months or beyond, and may depend on the availability of continuing rehabilitation treatment. Evolving concepts in neuroplasticity may offer hope for improved function years after the initial insult. Frequently, patients with mild residuae are left with minimal lower facial paresis, limited dexterity in the hand (e.g., diminished fine finger movements) and/or leg (e.g., diminished rate of toe tap), and/or foot drop.

3 *Ataxia.* Limb ataxia can occur with or without weakness and is a discoordination of movement usually related to infarction in the cerebellar hemisphere (**1.4**).[14] It is tested by evaluating rapid alternating movements and the finger-to-nose test in the upper extremities and the heel-to-shin test in the lower extremities. A midline cerebellar lesion may only cause mild vestibular symptoms and gait ataxia without limb involvement. Long-term recovery from ataxia is usually excellent.

4 *Sensory loss.* Sudden loss of sensation usually occurs in association with weakness in the same distribution, but pure hemibody sensory strokes can occur, usually from occlusions of small vessels supplying the lateral thalamus, pons, or lenticulocapsular region deep in the brain.[15–17] The patient usually describes numbness and/or tingling paresthesias on one side of the face or the hemibody, a feeling often likened to 'novocaine in the dentist's office' or 'having a limb fall asleep.'

Cortical lesions causing sensory deficits are further dichotomized into those of the insular and opercular areas, affecting primary (primitive) sensation of pain or temperature with intact position sense, versus those involving the postcentral gyrus, resulting in cortical sensory loss affecting position sense, stereognosis, and graphesthesia (**1.3B, 1.5**).[16]

Primary sensation is generally tested with a painful stimulus such as a pin-point or a stimulus of light touch, while cortical sensation may be assessed by testing position sense and by having a patient try to identify a number written upon the hand or an object placed into the hand. Inability to interpret the number written on the hand is **agraphesthesia** and an inability to identify an object such as a key in the hand is **astereognosis**.

Focal paresthesias, predominantly involving the perioral or finger areas (areas with strong representation within the homunculus), usually result from small distal emboli, to the postcentral gyrus (**1.5**).[16] Rarely, primitive sensory impairments evolve into dysesthesias, known as the **central post-stroke pain syndrome**.[16,18]

5 *Visual symptoms:*
- **Amaurosis fugax,** which is a term that describes transient blindness in one eye generally lasting 2–10 minutes, is a symptom of a retinal TIA often caused by an embolus from the ipsilateral carotid artery.[19,20] Permanent loss of vision in one eye frequently occurs when the central retinal artery is occluded, but this pattern of visual loss is generally not associated with other stroke symptoms (**1.6**).

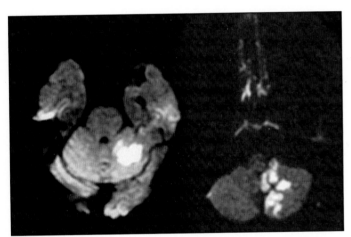

1.4 Ataxia. diffusion-weighted MRI sequences show (left) an acute infarct of the left cerebellar hemisphere, in the territory of the SCA, and (right) an infarct in the territory of the medial PICA.

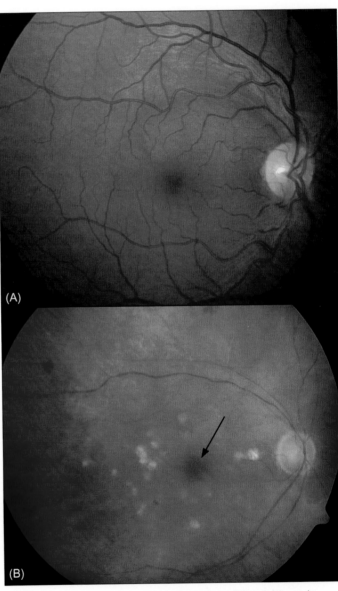

(A)

(B)

1.6 Monocular visual loss. A normal retina of the right eye is shown (A), contrasted with pallor and decreased vascularity due to acute central retinal artery occlusion (B). The diffuse whitening of the ischemic retina leaves only a 'cherry red spot' in the foveal center (arrow). (The small circular yellow spots are scars from past treatment of this retina with a laser.)

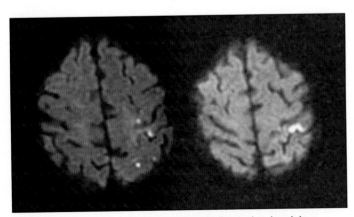

1.5 Cortical sensory loss. Cortical embolic stroke, involving the postcentral gyrus, caused a loss of cortical sensation. The emboli originated from atherosclerotic disease of the left ICA.

- **Hemifield visual loss** is loss of vision to one side involving both eyes.[21] It can be complete (hemianopia) or partial (quandrantanopia). It is detected by confrontational visual field testing in which the patient focuses on the examiner's nose and responds to stimuli in the fields of peripheral vision; it may be confirmed by computerized perimetry testing. Many patients with hemianopia are unaware of this symptom until demonstrated to them during their neurologic examination. Common presenting complaints are bumping into objects consistently on one side or, if driving, side-swiping a car present in the deficient visual hemifield. A stroke in the left hemisphere affecting the visual pathway will cause a right visual field defect, and vice versa. The further back the lesion is located in the visual pathway, the more homonymous (congruent) the defect in the two eyes (**1.7**). The chief practical results of a hemianopic visual field loss are that it usually precludes the ability to safely operate a motor vehicle and can make reading difficult. Spontaneous improvement of hemianopia typically occurs over the first 3 months post-stroke.[22]
- **Cortical blindness** is a rare clinical condition that results from infarction in both occipital lobes. The patient is blind but may describe visual phenomena. Anton's syndrome is the syndrome of cortical blindness in which patients deny their dense visual loss.[6]
- **Diplopia** (binocular double vision) may result from strokes in the posterior circulation because vertical and pontine gaze centers are located in the dorsal midbrain and pons, respectively (**1.8**).[6,23] The double images can

be horizontal, vertical, or oblique. Rarely, with brainstem stroke, the visual world may appear tilted.[6] When one eye is closed, there is no diplopia.
- **Forced gaze** to one side and gaze preference are important clinical findings in acute stroke.[6] Forced gaze means that both of the patient's eyes are deviated to one side and do not move from that position, a common early symptom in pontine strokes involving the horizontal gaze center. Gaze preference means that the patient's eyes are preferentially deviated in one direction but can be brought back to the midline or 'dolled' over to the contralateral side when the examiner moves the patient's head in the direction of the deviated eyes. These findings are consistent with a severe anterior circulation stroke involving the frontal eye fields on the same side as the gaze preference. For example, if the eyes are deviated to the right, one would expect a large stroke in the frontal region of the right hemisphere. The patient is said to be 'looking to the side of the stroke' (**1.9**).

6 *Visuospatial neglect.* Patients with infarction in the right (non-dominant) hemisphere are often unaware of the left side of the body or the left side of the space around them (**1.10**).[6,24] They do not recognize that the limbs on the left side are paralyzed or weak and are

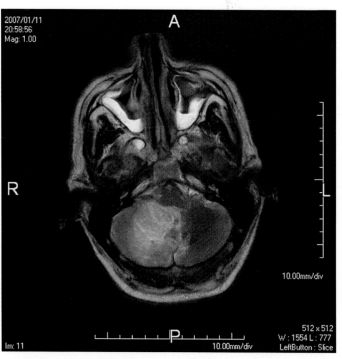

1.7 Hemifield visual loss. An acute infarct in the territory of the right PCA (arrowheads) on head CT scan (A) caused a left homonymous hemianopia. Other lesions, shown on a higher cut of this scan (B) in the right external capsule and the left posterior temporal lobe help explain this patient's vascular dementia.

1.8 Oculomotor impairment. Acute infarct of the right cerebellar hemisphere, with mass effect on the brainstem resulting in diploplia (T2-weighted MRI sequence).

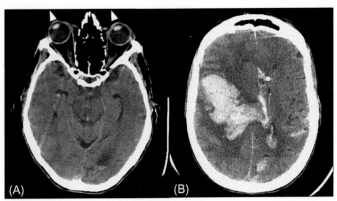

1.9 Gaze deviation. A patient with right gaze deviation (A). Note the far right position of the lenses of the eyes (arrowheads) on a lower cut of the CT scan. The responsible lesion, a large right frontoparietal intracerebral hemorrhage (B), impaired the patient's ability to drive the eyes to the left, a function of the right frontal eye fields.

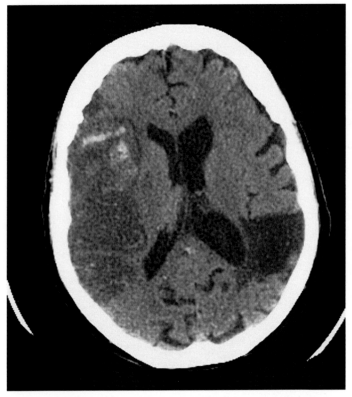

1.10 Hemineglect. Head CT scan demonstrates a subacute right hemispheric stroke that caused left body hemineglect. The evolving right hemispheric edema causes mass effect on the adjacent right lateral ventricle, while a chronic, left MCA infarct caused atrophy and associated *ex-vacuo* enlargement of the left lateral ventricle.

often unable to identify their left body parts; the patient may deny ownership of a paretic limb. Most commonly due to right parietal infarction, this inability to recognize a deficit is called **anosagnosia**. In a milder form, when presented with visual or sensory stimuli to both sides of the body at the same time (bilateral simultaneous stimuli), patients may 'extinguish' (not perceive) the stimulus on the left. Hemineglect is a predictor for poor rehabilitation and functional outcomes post-stroke.[25,26]

7 *Language and speech production:*
- **Dysarthria** is slurring or mispronunciation of normal speech. The words and sentences are correct, but the patient may be difficult to understand. Dysarthria can be heard in patients with facial or tongue weakness and also occurs in strokes involving the cerebellum and brainstem. Patients often state that they are 'speaking like they were drunk.'
- **Aphasia** is difficulty with language processing: production and/or comprehension of speech. The stroke responsible occurs in the dominant (usually left) hemisphere.
  - *Broca's aphasia* (expressive and non-fluent) is a condition in which the patient has difficulty with naming and has very halted, frustrated, effortful speech. There is no difficulty understanding spoken language. The patient may state: 'I knew what I wanted to say, but just couldn't find the words.' Broca's area is an anatomical site at the base of the motor strip in the dominant hemisphere (**1.3B, 1.11A,B**). This type of aphasia is often associated with contralateral limb (arm > leg) and facial weakness.
  - *Wernicke's aphasia* (receptive and fluent) is a condition in which the patient cannot understand spoken language, but talks 'fluently' in long sentences often devoid of nouns and most meaning. Wernicke's area is an anatomical site near the angular gyrus in the dominant hemisphere (**1.3B, 1.11C**). Wernicke's aphasia may exist without motor impairment, and thus, the patient may be misdiagnosed as being simply 'confused,' or 'intoxicated.'
  - *Global aphasia* is the condition where the patient has both expressive and receptive deficits. Patients are frequently mute, and must rely upon visual mimicry to follow along with a neurologic exam.

Aphasia resulting from stroke will frequently evolve and usually improve, such that its basic characteristics fluctuate. Patients often will describe that their fluency will seem to break down when they are tired at the end of a long day. Subtle improvements in language-related deficits may occur even months to years following a stroke.

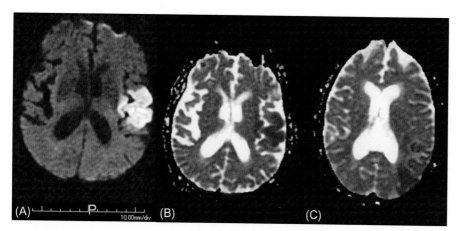

1.11 Aphasia. A diffusion-weighted MRI sequence (A) and apparent diffusion coefficient map (B) of a left MCA lesion, involving an anterior branch and affecting predominantly the insular cortex clinically expressed as Broca's (non-fluent, expressive) aphasia. A second acute left MCA infarct, apparent diffusion coefficient map (C) clinically associated with Wernicke's (fluent, receptive) aphasia.

8 *Cognitive and behavioral deficits.* Although aphasia and neglect are the most common higher cognitive deficits related to stroke, a wider range of neurobehavioral deficits include apraxia, memory loss and dementia, fatigue, depression, and other psychiatric disorders (e.g., emotional incontinence, anger, anxiety) can occur.[6,27] Given the advancing age of the general population, strong interest has arisen in the field of cognitive/neurobehavioral deficits associated with stroke. Large-scale clinical trials have begun to investigate vascular dementia resulting from multiple ischemic infarctions (e.g., **1.7**) and post-stroke depression.[28,29]

Stroke outcomes

An excellent predictor of stroke outcomes is stroke severity at presentation. A measure of stroke-related neurologic deficits, the National Institutes of Health Stroke Scale (NIHSS) score has been extensively studied in clinical trials and has been shown to be a very useful predictor of 3-month outcomes. NIHSS scores from 0 to 10 (mild deficits); 11 to 20 (moderate); and >20 (severe) have decreasing potential for good outcomes (*Table 1.3*).[30] The NIHSS is an excellent way for clinicians to communicate the severity of a stroke. Physicians and nurses caring for patients with strokes can be certified in the use of the NIHSS by the American Stroke Association or the National Stroke Association on their respective websites. Training materials can be obtained from the National Institutes of Neurologic Disease and Stroke (NINDS) website. The NIHSS score is heavily weighted toward anterior-circulation strokes, such that aphasia and hemiparesis often account for most of the points accumulated by any individual patient. Posterior circulation strokes frequently include neurologic

signs such as nystagmus, dysmetria, gait imbalance, or dysarthria, which do not contribute significantly to the NIHSS score, such that the score may underestimate the severity of a posterior circulation lesion.[31] In addition, a left middle cerebral artery stroke will have a higher NIHSS than an equally severe right middle cerebral artery stroke because of the scoring for language impairment. In practice, it is relatively simple to indicate to patients and their families how severe the deficit appears to be based solely upon the neurologic examination and NIHSS score. The potential for good outcomes is poor in moderate to severe strokes if left untreated.

Other common types of outcomes scales measure different dimensions of recovery and disability after acute stroke.[31] Some were developed specifically for stroke patients, while others look at disability and recovery following any type of acute brain injury:

Table 1.3 Admission NIHSS Score predicts short-term outcomes from acute ischemic stroke*

PROACT-II. Percentage of patients with minimal or no deficits (Modified Rankin Scale, 0–1), at 90 days post-stroke:

NIHSS 4–10: 63%

NIHSS 11–20: 24%

NIHSS 21–30: 7%

Adapted from Furlan *et al.*[37]

TOAST

NIHSS ≤6: 80% Excellent or good outcome

NIHSS ≥16: >85% Severe disability or death

Adapted from Adams *et al.*[30]

*Data derived from control groups' outcomes in two clinical trials, PROACT-II and TOAST.

- *Barthel Index (BI)* assesses activities of self-care and mobility.
- *Modified Rankin Scale (mRS)* assesses functional independence.
- *Glasgow Outcome Scale (GOS)* assesses general level of disability and recovery following acute brain injury.
- *PHQ-9[32]* assesses depression.
- *Stroke-specific Quality of Life scale[33]* assesses quality of life.

The National Institute of Neurological Disorders and Stroke Recombinant Tissue Plasminogen Activator (NINDS rt-PA) Stroke Trial combined the NIHSS, mRS, BI, and GOS into a single global outcomes measure.[34] Most acute stroke clinical trials use the mRS at 90 days as a primary outcome measure.

Diagnosis of stroke

The diagnosis of stroke is made by taking a careful history, performing a neurologic examination, and confirming the clinical diagnosis with an appropriate neuroimaging study. Seizures, hypoglycemia, trauma, and migraine are the most common mimics of the focal neurologic deficits in acute stroke. Brain tumors occasionally present with sudden onset of symptoms due to an associated hemorrhage into the tumor. Global symptoms of stroke such as altered level of conscious can be mimicked by metabolic encephalopathy. In most cases, the clinical diagnosis of stroke is not difficult. However, patients with global encephalopathy due to diagnoses such as venous sinus thrombosis, vasculitis, or multifocal emboli are more challenging; these cases are usually diagnosed by neuroimaging.

Neuroimaging

The evolution of modern neuroimaging has revolutionized the diagnosis and management of stroke. The modalities currently used are listed here and will be shown throughout the text.

- Non-enhanced head computed tomography (CT) scans are the most commonly available neuroimaging studies for acute stroke. This modality is excellent in detecting ICH and SAH (**1.1C,E**, **1.9B**), but is insensitive to small areas of infarction, especially in the posterior fossa (**1.12**). In most cases of early infarction (e.g., 1–4 hours after onset), the CT scan is normal. Subsequent scans over the next few hours begin to demonstrate an evolving infarct (**1.13**).
- Well-delineated hypodensity on CT indicates infarcted tissue (**1.13C**).

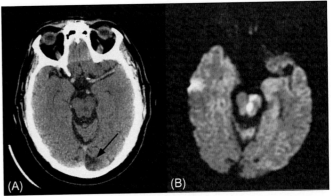

1.12 Paramedian pontine stroke. (A) Non-contrast head CT scan shows a faint hypodensity in mid-pons. The hypodense lesion in the left occipital pole (arrow) is likely a small, old PCA stroke. (B) The diffusion-weighted MRI study readily delineates the acute stroke as an area of restricted diffusion in the left medial pons.

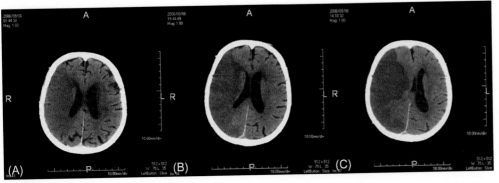

1.13 Serial neuroimaging, infarct in evolution. A right MCA-territory AIS on head CT scans. (A) Note blurring of sulcal spaces, and early hypodensity, at 6 hours. (B) The hypodense lesion becomes better delineated, at 24 hours. (C) The lesion demarcated as a wide hypodensity, with mass effect along the midline, at 40 hours.

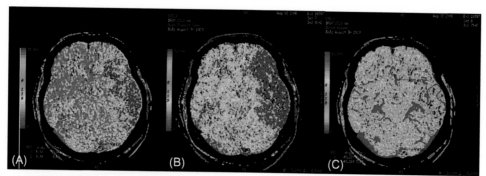

1.14 Perfusion CT imaging. (A) Cerebral blood flow map: hypoperfusion in a wide left-MCA distribution. (B) Mean transit time map: the region of slow mean transit time mirrors that of the cerebral blood flow map. (C) Cerebral blood volume map: no significant region of low volume is observed, suggesting that this ischemic tissue has not as yet infarcted. This cerebral blood flow/cerebral blood volume mismatch is consistent with an ischemic penumbra that might benefit from reperfusion therapy.[35]

- CT angiography using iodinated contrast dye can be used in the acute setting to diagnose large vessel extracranial and intracranial occlusions, and provides outstanding resolution for assessing the morphology of intracranial aneurysms and their position relative to the skull base.
- CT perfusion studies can delineate a region of decreased cerebral blood flow, and may be combined with other imaging modalities to identify hypoperfused 'tissue-at-risk' for infarction. If the area of decreased cerebral blood flow 'matches' the area of very low cerebral blood volume then that area will typically go on to infarct (**1.14**). If the area of decreased cerebral blood volume is quite small compared with the area of decreased cerebral blood flow (mismatch), reperfusion treatment

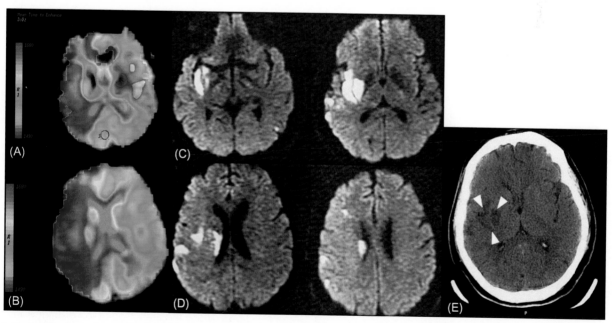

1.15 Perfusion–diffusion mismatch. This 52-year-old patient with a history of hypertension and tobacco use presented with acute-onset left hemiplegia, and a head CT scan (not shown) with a hyperdense middle cerebral artery sign, consistent with a proximal MCA occlusion. The perfusion-weighted MRI scan, here a map of mean transit time (A,B), shows deficient blood flow throughout the right MCA territory as a red region, but the diffusion-weighted MRI sequence (C,D) shows a smaller area of patchy infarction. This perfusion–diffusion mismatch directed reperfusion therapy, and the good outcome was confirmed with a follow-up CT scan 1 day later demonstrating only a small, predominantly subcortical infarct as a hypodense lesion (arrowheads) (E).

may prevent infarction. The mean transit time also has predictive value.[35]

- Magnetic resonance imaging (MRI) is not as readily available for acute stroke diagnosis in many hospitals. The diffusion-weighted image sequence is sensitive to ischemia within minutes of the onset of symptoms (**1.4, 1.15**). This technique is helpful when the diagnosis is in question and is excellent for identifying very small strokes causing minimal neurologic deficits. A 'dark' or hypointense lesion on the apparent diffusion coefficient map confirms that a diffusion-weighted magnetic resonance imaging lesion is due to infarction (**1.11**).

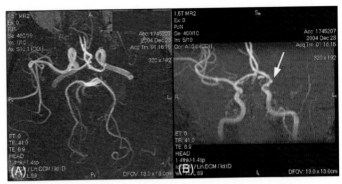

1.16 Magnetic resonance angiography, intracranial study. Proximal occlusion of the left middle cerebral artery, the M1 segment, on coronal (A) and transaxial (B) views (arrow). No distal, left hemispheric blood flow is observed.

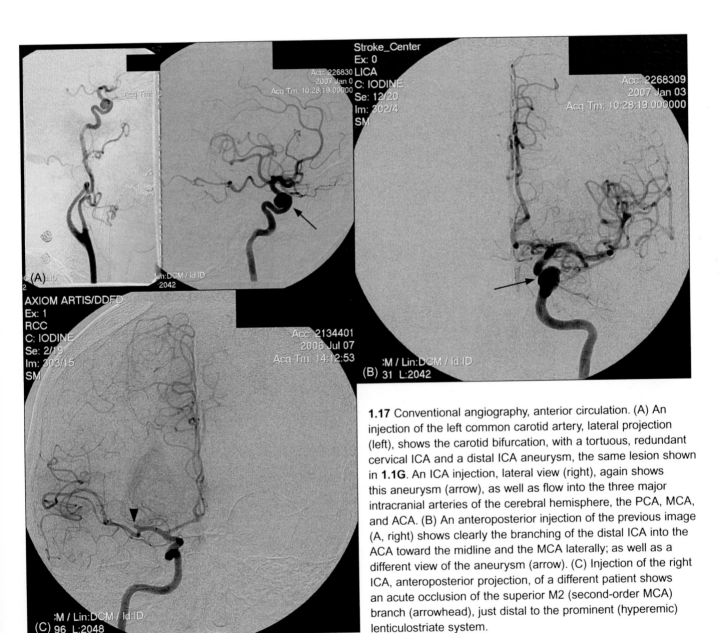

1.17 Conventional angiography, anterior circulation. (A) An injection of the left common carotid artery, lateral projection (left), shows the carotid bifurcation, with a tortuous, redundant cervical ICA and a distal ICA aneurysm, the same lesion shown in **1.1G**. An ICA injection, lateral view (right), again shows this aneurysm (arrow), as well as flow into the three major intracranial arteries of the cerebral hemisphere, the PCA, MCA, and ACA. (B) An anteroposterior injection of the previous image (A, right) shows clearly the branching of the distal ICA into the ACA toward the midline and the MCA laterally; as well as a different view of the aneurysm (arrow). (C) Injection of the right ICA, anteroposterior projection, of a different patient shows an acute occlusion of the superior M2 (second-order MCA) branch (arrowhead), just distal to the prominent (hyperemic) lenticulostriate system.

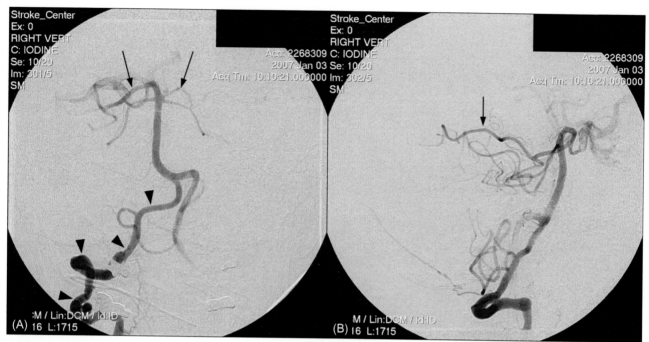

1.18 Conventional angiography, posterior circulation. (A) A right vertebral artery (arrowheads) injection, anteroposterior view, shows the major intracranial arteries of the posterior circulation. The SCAs course immediately below and almost parallel to the PCAs (arrows). (B) A lateral view of the image in (A) shows a slightly later time-frame of this injection, with the PCA (arrow) at the top of the BA extending posteriorly toward the occipital lobe.

- When there is a small area of abnormality in the diffusion-weighted image sequence and a large area of abnormality in the perfusion-weighted sequence, there is a so-called 'perfusion/diffusion mismatch' (**1.15**),[36] which is akin to the cerebral blood flow/cerebral blood volume findings of perfusion CT imaging. A mismatch indicates an opportunity to salvage tissue that is underperfused but not yet showing a diffusion deficit indicating cellular injury. This kind of physiologic analysis may be the best way to predict which cases could tolerate a longer time window for intravenous reperfusion therapy and/or those who should go on to neurointervention.
- Magnetic resonance angiography is useful in screening for extracranial and intracranial large vessel occlusions or stenoses (**1.16**). In general, magnetic resonance angiography tends to overestimate the degree of stenosis, but gadolinium, a contrast agent, improves the quality of this technique.
- Digital subtraction angiography, also called conventional cerebral angiography (**1.17**, **1.18**), is the gold standard for visualization of extracranial and intracranial vessels, but has the disadvantage of being invasive and requiring specialized equipment, technicians, and interventional neuroradiologists.

References

1. Johnston S. Transient ischemic attack. *N Engl J Med* 2002; **347**: 1687–92.
2. UN Chronicle Health Watch. *Atlas of Heart Disease and Stroke*. 2005; **0105**: 46.
3. Warlow C, Sudlow C, Dennis M, Wardlaw J, Sandercock P. Stroke. *Lancet* 2003; **362**: 1211–24.
4. Reddy K, Yusuf S. Emerging epidemic of cardiovascular disease in developing countries. *Circulation* 1998; **97**: 596–601.
5. Albers G, Amarenco P, Easton J, Sacco R, Teal P. Antithrombotic and thrombolytic therapy for ischemic stroke: The Seventh ACCP Conference on Antithrombotic and Thrombolytic Therapy. *Chest* 2004; **3**: S483–512.
6. Brazis P, Masdeu J, Biller J. *Localization in Clinical Neurology*, 4th edn. Philadelphia: Lippincott Williams & Wilkins; 2001.

7. Bogousslavsky J, Hommel M. Ischemic stroke syndromes: clinical features, anatomy, vascular territories. In: Adams H, Jr, ed. *Handbook of Cerebrovascular Diseases*. New York: Marcel Dekker; 1993: 51–94.

8. Bogousslavsky J, Caplan L. *Stroke Syndromes*, 2nd edn. New York: Cambridge University Press; 2001.

9. Estol C. Headache: stroke symptoms and signs. In: Bogousslavsky J, Caplan L, eds. *Stroke Syndromes*, 2nd edn. New York: Cambridge University Press; 2001: 60–75.

10. Schievink W. Spontaneous dissection of the carotid and vertebral arteries. *N Engl J Med* 2001; **344**: 898–906.

11. Pinho e Melo T, Bogousslavsky J. Hemiparesis and other types of motor weakness. In: Bogousslavsky J, Caplan L, eds. *Stroke Syndromes*, 2nd edn. New York: Cambridge University Press; 2001: 22–33.

12. Goldstein L, Bertels C, Davis J. Interrater reliability of the NIH stroke scale. *Arch Neurol* 1989; **46**: 660–2.

13. Dobkin B. Rehabilitation after stroke. *N Engl J Med* 2005; **352**: 1677–84.

14. Timmann D, Diener H. Cerebellar ataxia. In: Bogousslavsky J, Caplan L, eds. *Stroke Syndromes*, 2nd edn. New York: Cambridge University Press; 2001: 48–59.

15. Kim J. Sensory abnormality. In: Bogousslavsky J, Caplan L, eds. *Stroke Syndromes*, 2nd edn. New York: Cambridge University Press; 2001.

16. Kim J. Patterns of sensory abnormality in cortical stroke: evidence for a dichotomized sensory system. *Neurology* 2007; **68**: 174–80.

17. Schmahmann J. Vascular syndromes of the thalamus. *Stroke* 2003; **34**: 2264–78.

18. Bowsher D, Leijon G, Thuomas K-A. Central poststroke pain: correlation of MRI with clinical pain characteristics and sensory abnormalities. *Neurology* 1998; **51**: 1352–8.

19. Benavente O, Eliasziw M, Streifler J, *et al.* Prognosis after transient monocular blindness associated with carotid-artery stenosis. *N Engl J Med* 2001; **345**: 1084–90.

20. Wray S. Visual symptoms (eye). In: Bogousslavsky J, Caplan L, eds. *Stroke Syndromes*, 2nd edn. New York: Cambridge University Press; 2001: 111–28.

21. Barton J, Caplan L. Cerebral visual dysfunction. In: Bogousslavsky J, Caplan L, eds. *Stroke Syndromes*, 2nd edn. New York: Cambridge University Press; 2001: 87–110.

22. Zhang X, Kedar S, Lynn M, Newman N, Biousse V. Natural history of homonymous hemianopia. *Neurology* 2006; **66**: 901–5.

23. Pierrot-Deseilligny C. Eye movement abnormalities. In: Bogousslavsky J, Caplan L, eds. *Stroke Syndromes*, 2nd edn. New York: Cambridge University Press; 2001: 76–86.

24. Clarke S. Right hemisphere syndromes. In: Bogousslavsky J, Caplan L, eds. *Stroke Syndromes*, 2nd edn. New York: Cambridge University Press; 2001: 264–72.

25. Beis J-M, Keller C, Morin N, *et al.* Right spatial neglect after left hemisphere stroke: a qualitative and quantitative study. *Neurology* 2004; **63**: 1600–5.

26. Buxbaum L, Ferraro M, Veramonti T, *et al.* Hemispatial neglect: subtypes, neuroanatomy, and disability. *Neurology* 2004; **62**: 749–56.

27. Bogousslavsky J. William Feinberg Lecture 2002: emotions, mood, and behavior after stroke. *Stroke* 2003; **34**: 1046–50.

28. Hackett M, Anderson C, House A. Management of depression after stroke: a systematic review of pharmacological therapies. *Stroke* 2005; **36**: 1092–7.

29. Erkinjuntti T, Roman G, Gauthier S, Feldman H, Rockwood K. Emerging therapies for vascular dementia and vascular cognitive impairment. *Stroke* 2004; **35**: 1010–17.

30. Adams HP Jr, Davis P, Leira E, *et al.* Baseline NIH Stroke Scale score strongly predicts outcome after stroke: a report of the Trial of Org 10172 in Acute Stroke Treatment (TOAST). *Neurology* 1999; **53**: 126–31.

31. Kasner S. Clinical interpretation and use of stroke scales. *Lancet Neurol* 2006; **5**: 603–12.

32. Williams L, Brizendine E, Plue L, *et al.* Performance of the PHQ-9 as a screening tool for depression after stroke. *Stroke* 2005; **36**: 635–8.

33. Williams L, Weinberger M, Harris L, Clark D, Biller J. Development of a stroke-specific quality of life scale. *Stroke* 1999; **30**: 1362–9.

34. National Institute of Neurological Disorders and Stroke rt-PA Stroke Study Group. Tissue plasminogen activator for acute ischemic stroke. *N Engl J Med* 1995; **333**: 1581–7.

35. Wintermark M, Reichart M, Thiran J-P, *et al*. Prognostic accuracy of cerebral blood flow measurement by perfusion computed tomography, at the time of emergency room admission in acute stroke patients. *Ann Neurol* 2002; 51: 417–32.

36. Davalos A, Blanco M, Pedraza S, *et al*. The clinical–DWI mismatch: A new diagnostic approach to the brain tissue at risk of infarction. *Neurology* 2004; **62**: 2187–92.

37. Furlan A, Higashida R, Katzan I, Abou–Chebl A. Intra-arterial thrombolysis in acute ischemic stroke. In: Lyden P, ed. *Thrombolytic Therapy for Stroke*. Totowa, NJ: Humana Press; 2001: 175–95.

Further reading

Bogousslavsky J, Caplan LR. *Stroke Syndromes*, 2nd edn. New York: Cambridge University Press; 2001.

Brazis PW, Masdeu JC, Biller J. *Localization in Clinical Neurology*, 4th edn. New York: Little, Brown and Company; 2001.

Kasner S. Clinical interpretation and use of stroke scales. *Lancet Neurol* 2006; **5**: 603–12.

Resources for patients

American Stroke Association: http://www.strokeassociation.org

National Stroke Association: http://www.stroke.org

Therapies: The Management of Acute Ischemic Stroke and Secondary Stroke Prevention

Introduction

The rapidly evolving and increasing ability to treat AIS effectively is one of the most exciting topics in medicine. Acute stroke treatment is time-dependent so it is important to stress the need for stroke victims to reach the hospitals most able to offer the best combination of drug and device treatment(s). This means that regional stroke networks and efficient transfer processes will be key to increasing the number of people treated. This chapter addresses the state of acute treatments and secondary prevention for ischemic stroke.

Overview

Key variables influencing the viability of brain tissue during AIS include: **time, hemodynamics, tissue**, and **intervention** (*Table 2.1*).[1] Most of the effort to improve outcomes in ischemic stroke has focused on decreasing the time to treatment and pharmacologic or mechanical interventions for reperfusion or neuroprotection. More sophisticated assessment of hemodynamic issues, particularly collateral circulation, may influence what interventions are recommended at what point in time. Maximizing tissue viability through tight control of serum glucose and hypothermia is being evaluated.

The challenges of providing optimal treatment for every patient to improve clinical outcomes are significant:

1 *Time*. Although the healthcare systems in many countries are evolving to address acute stroke as a highest-level medical emergency, public awareness of stroke symptoms remains low. If stroke symptoms are not recognized or patients not rapidly transported to 'stroke-ready' hospitals, then any efforts to develop treatments to improve stroke outcomes during the critical initial minutes-to-hours will be wasted. In the USA, Emergency Medical Services (EMS) are organized at the community and/ or state-wide level making the early response to acute stroke patients highly variable. Benchmarks for hospital performance have been established to encourage rapid treatment on arrival.[2] The recommended time from door-to-computed tomography (CT) scan is 25 minutes, and from door-to-drug (intravenous (IV) tissue plasminogen activator (t-PA)) 60 minutes.

2 *Healthcare resources*. The capacity of individual hospitals to care for acute stroke varies widely. In the USA, national and regional quality improvement initiatives have led to formal certification/identification of acute 'stroke-ready' medical centers;[3] however, many hospitals lack adequate infrastructure and medical staff to meet all of the needs of acute stroke patients. Most likely, a two-tiered system will emerge with Primary Stroke Centers capable of rapid triage and administration of IV thrombolysis partnering with regional Comprehensive Stroke Centers that offer subspecialty neurovascular care, clinical trials, physician training programs, and endovascular (IA) treatments. The Joint Commission began certifying Primary Stroke Centers in the USA in 2004, and criteria for Comprehensive Stroke Centers have been published.[4]

3 *Stroke clinical trials*. The modern era of acute stroke clinical trials is in its infancy in regard to drug and device development and clinical trial design. Patient selection and outcomes can be based on clinical criteria alone or may include neuroimaging criteria. The pathophysiologic heterogeneity of stroke makes the assessment of outcomes even more challenging.[5]

Table 2.1 Factors for tissue viability in acute ischemic stroke

1. Time
- Acute Stroke Team, protocols → reduce time-to-treatment
- Public awareness → use of '911' EMS systems
- *Impact*: speed time to starting acute therapies

2. Hemodynamics
- *Collateral circulation*: circle of Willis; leptomeningeal
- Extracranial and intracranial stenoses
- *Measure*: neuroimaging to define, perfusion CT/MRI studies
- *Impact*: manipulate systemic blood pressure, acute occlusive lesions

3. Tissue
- Local metabolic, hemostatic, vascular, structural changes secondary to ischemia
- *Measure*: age, gender, serum glucose, temperature, blood pressure, oxygenation
- *Impact*: correcting treatable variables that may impact upon brain tissue viability (e.g., hyperthermia, hyperglycemia, coagulability)

4. Intervention
- Reperfusion tactics, neuro/cytoprotection
- *Impact*: IV/IA thrombolysis, devices for vessel recanalization

Adapted from Warach.[1]

4 *Complexity of cerebral ischemia.* Understanding of the biology of cerebral ischemia, which is the basis for new drug and device development, continues to evolve. The time-dependent cascade of acute focal ischemia is illustrated (**2.1**).[6] Drugs that interrupt or slow the ischemic cascade may interact with only one of the various steps. Ischemia affects not only neurons (constituting <5% of the cells in cerebral gray matter) but also astrocytes and other glial cells supporting neurons, the axons of neurons (which relay signals to other cells), and the microvessels that supply oxygen and nutrients.[7] Treatments that target this entire 'neurovascular unit' rather than simply neurons may be more effective in treating acute ischemic brain injury (**2.2**).[7]

Treatment for acute ischemic stroke

The modern era of treatments for AIS was ushered in by clinical trials that began in the 1980s and early 1990s. Two major therapeutic approaches have been studied since the early trials were conducted:

- **Reperfusion treatments** include IV or IA drugs and endovascular devices aimed at the recanalization of occluded intracranial and extracranial arteries. IV t-PA was approved for the treatment of AIS within 3 hours of onset of symptoms in the USA in 1996.[8] The Merci Retriever® was approved for the removal of clots from intracranial and extracranial cerebral arteries within 8 hours of stroke symptoms onset in 2004 (**2.3; case study 1**).[9] A second endovascular thrombectomy device, the Penumbra Stroke System, was similarly approved by the Food and Drug Administration (FDA) in 2008 for its aspiration mechanism.[10]
- **Neuroprotective agents** or devices are meant to maintain optimal tissue viability in the ischemic penumbra. No pharmacologic agent has been shown to be effective. Trials of hypothermia and infrared laser to test potential for neuroprotection are currently in progress.[11]
- The scope of established and putative treatments for AIS is shown in *Table 2.2*.[11] The stage is set for an explosion in treatment modalities during the upcoming decades.[6,7,12]

Reperfusion treatment and time

Time is brain! For every minute stroke is left untreated, an estimated 1.9 million neurons are destroyed.[13] The benefit of IV t-PA has been demonstrated to wane through the 3-hour window.[14] However, subsequent pooled analysis of three major clinical trials suggests that the time window of effectiveness for IV t-PA may actually be as long as 4.5 hours.[15] Recent clinical trials evidence from the European study group subsequently went on to prove that IV t-PA is efficacious for AIS within this 3 to 4.5-hour time window.[16]

IA treatments, initially catheter-delivered thrombolytic agents, such as pro-urokinase[17,18] directly address the arterial clot responsible for AIS. In addition to drugs, the catheter itself and other devices such as balloon angioplasty, flexible stents, and clot retrieval devices can be used to manipulate thrombus and recanalize vessels. Successful outcomes with IA treatment may occur well beyond the traditional 3-hour

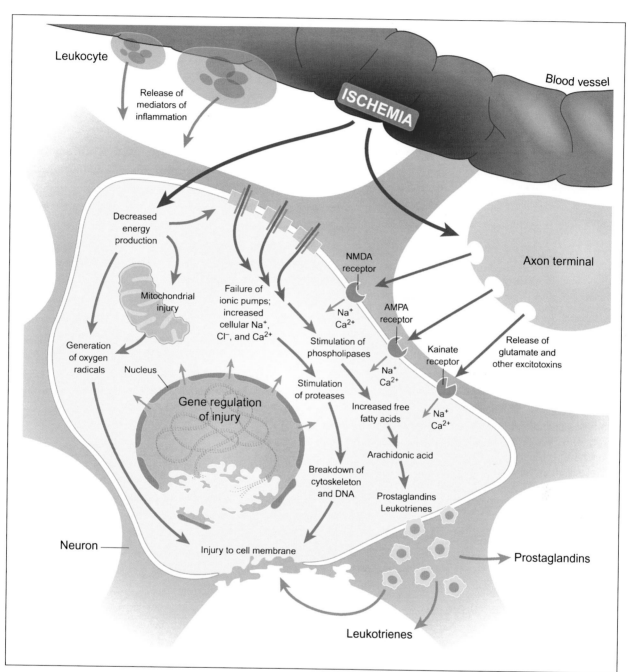

2.1 The molecular events initiated in brain tissue by acute cerebral ischemia. Interruption of cerebral blood flow results in decreased energy production, which in turn causes failure of ionic pumps, mitochondrial injury, activation of leukocytes (with release of mediators of inflammation), generation of oxygen radicals, and release of excitotoxins. Increased cellular levels of sodium, chloride, and calcium ions result in stimulation of phospholipases and proteases, followed by generation and release of prostaglandins and leukotrienes, breakdown of DNA and the cytoskeleton, and ultimately, breakdown of the cell membrane. Alteration of genetic components regulates elements of the cascade to alter the degree of injury. AMPA denotes α-amino-3-hydroxy-5-methyl-4-isoxazole propionic acid and NMDA *N*-methyl-ᴅ-aspartate. Adapted with permission from Brott *et al.*[6]

time window for IV t-PA. Timeframes of 6–8 hours for anterior circulation strokes and 12–48 hours for posterior circulation strokes have been reported in case series and formal clinical trials.[12]

The two leading endovascular approaches are IA thrombolysis and the Merci Retriever® (**case study 1**). IA thrombolysis has limited randomized clinical trial data to support its efficacy.[18,19] Current guidelines recommend IA

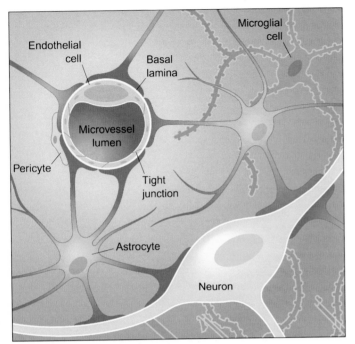

2.2 The neurovascular unit. A conceptual framework, the neurovascular unit is comprised of neurons, the microvessels that supply them, and their supporting cells. Cerebral microvessels consist of the endothelium (which forms the blood–brain barrier), the basal lamina matrix, and the end-feet of astrocytes. Microglial cells and pericytes may also participate in the unit. Communication has been shown to occur between neurons and microvessels through astrocytes. Adapted from del Zoppo.[7]

thrombolysis for selected patients who have major stroke of <6 hours duration due to occlusions of the MCA and who are otherwise not candidates for IV t-PA and for patients with contraindications (e.g., recent surgery) to the use of IV thrombolysis;[20] however, criteria for patient selection and evaluation of optimal IA treatments are subjects of ongoing investigation.[19]

The potential advantages of IA thrombolysis over IV t-PA include: direct angiographic visualization of the lesion responsible for AIS; the ability to mechanically disrupt the thrombus with guidewire and catheter; improved recanalization rates for selected proximal lesions of higher thrombus burden (e.g., basilar,[21] proximal MCA,[22] and distal ICA occlusions[23]); lower dose of thrombolytic agent (e.g., 5–20 mg IA t-PA, versus a maximal IV t-PA dose of 90 mg); and the longer time windows. The Merci Retriever® also enables direct analysis of the pathogenesis of AIS, when thromboembolic material is retrieved for pathologic study (**2.3**).[9,24] The potential barriers to the widespread use of endovascular approaches are their limited availability at acute care hospitals in most countries and the additional time, often 1–2 hours, to prepare such interventional procedures.

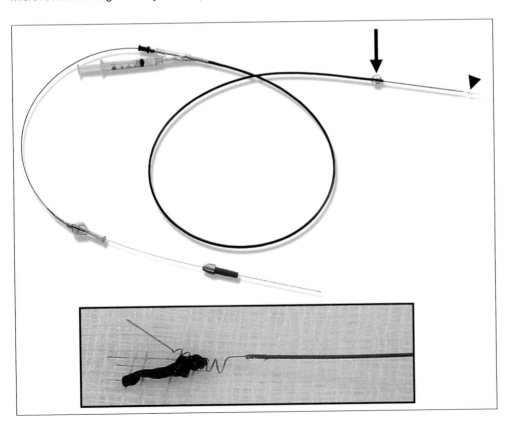

2.3 The Merci Retriever®.[9] The earlier-generation clot retrieval device consists of a flexible helical snare (arrowhead) that uncoils beyond and into the thrombo-occlusive lesion (see inset), and a balloon (arrow) that enables proximal protection, to prevent blood flow from fragmenting and embolizing the ensnared clot up into the cerebral vasculature. Image published with permission, courtesy of Concentric Medical, Inc.

Table 2.2 Therapeutic modalities for reperfusion therapy during acute ischemic stroke

Fibrinolytic agents
- Established: IV t-PA
- Novel, experimental: tenecteplase, desmoteplase, reteplase, microplasmin

Glycoprotein IIb/IIIa antagonists
- Abciximab, tirofiban

Combined pharmacological approaches
a. Lytics and antithrombotics
  (i)   Examples (in preliminary trials): IV t-PA + tirofiban; reteplase + abciximab; eptifibatide + t-PA; argatroban (direct thrombin inhibitor) + t-PA
b. Lytics and neuroprotectants
  (i)   Hypothermia
  (ii) Magnesium (in field), with in-hospital reperfusion
c. Lytics and vasoprotectants
  (i)   NXY-059 (spin trap agent) ± IV t-PA
d. Sonothrombolysis
  (i)   2-MHz continuous ultrasound monitoring + t-PA

Endovascular mechanical treatments
- Intra-arterial fibrinolysis
- Mechanical disruption of occlusive material
- Endovascular thrombectomy

Note: The above list includes drugs and devices that have been trialed, rejected, and/or approved in clinical studies. t-PA, tissue plasminogen activator.
Adapted from Molina *et al.*[12]

Combination modalities

Some of the combined modalities for treatment studied to date are listed in *Table 2.2*. The development of multimodal approaches combining drugs and devices is not dissimilar from those employed for acute coronary syndromes.[11,25] Key challenges with acute pharmacologic and endovascular interventions in the brain versus the heart are: (1) greater technical difficulty in accessing intracranial arteries with endovascular devices due to smaller, more tortuous vessels; (2) the susceptibility to reperfusion hemorrhage in the brain; and (3) limited accessibility to interventional specialists to perform endovascular procedures for AIS. In the USA, for example, hundreds of hospitals are capable of performing IA treatments for acute coronary syndromes, while only a few dozen are well-staffed with neurointerventionalists to treat AIS around the clock.

Neuroimaging

Modern neuroimaging has revolutionized acute stroke treatment by helping clinicians to more accurately and rapidly select patients best suited for emergent interventions.

Multimodal MRI and CT imaging protocols, developed only in the past decade, help identify patients most likely to benefit from reperfusion and direct treatments based on lesion-specific data. Neuroimaging differentiates AIS from acute hemorrhage, detects very early ischemia, quantifies and delineates irreversibly infarcted core tissue from salvageable penumbra, demonstrates areas of hemorrhagic transformation, and identifies large vessel occlusions and stenoses. All of this information can be rapidly obtained in 5–20 minutes.[12] The resultant data indicate the degree of collateral circulation, a critical variable in eventual infarct size. Strong collateral circulation (direct, via the circle of Willis, and indirect, via adjacent leptomeningeal supply) can keep a large area of penumbral tissue viable for an extended period of time, while patients with poor collaterals are less likely to do well even with early recanalization. The neuroimaging data enable patient selection based upon an individualized, physiologic 'tissue clock' rather than a fixed chronologic clock.[12]

The concept of the 'mismatch model' discussed in Chapter 1 to assess areas of brain viability based on perfusion MRI and CT techniques is gaining credibility. In this model, a core (irreversible) infarct is surrounded by a region of salvageable ischemic penumbra, and an adjacent region of benign oligemia.[26] Modern clinical trials have begun to incorporate real-time neuroimaging data into their patient selection and outcomes data. Current research is utilizing functional MRI and CT imaging in an effort to select patients with viable ischemic tissue who could benefit from recanalization beyond 3 hours. These newer neuroradiologic techniques may identify those patients who may be assisted by reperfusion and other treatments as well as those who cannot be helped (**case study 2**) and who could even potentially be harmed.

Management of acute ischemic stroke

Acute stroke is 'brain shock.' The part of the brain that is affected lacks blood supply and, therefore, oxygen and glucose. The goal is to reperfuse as quickly as possible and resuscitate 'shocked (stunned) brain.' Guidelines on the standard of care for patients with AIS are published periodically by the American Stroke Association (*Table 2.3*).[20] Ample clinical trials evidence also has demonstrated that stroke patients' outcomes are improved with care in dedicated stroke units, largely by averting post-stroke medical complications (e.g., deep vein thrombosis, aspiration).[27]

In cases of massive hemispheric stroke, most typically involving the entire territory of the MCA, the development of malignant edema results in herniation syndromes with high early mortality rates. Hemicraniectomy (removal of the skull on one side of the head, with duraplasty) is sometimes recommended as a life-saving tactic (**case study 3**).[28] Recently, a pooled analysis of three randomized controlled European trials documented a strong benefit of this approach in patients <60 years of age with malignant MCA territory infarction.[29] Patients with large infarcts of the cerebellar hemisphere, usually in the territory of the posterior inferior cerebellar artery, may similarly face a high early mortality from brainstem compression, yet also have encouraging outcomes with surgical decompression of the posterior fossa.

It is likely that acute stroke treatment will always be time-dependent, with the best outcomes resulting from the earliest interventions paired with meticulous medical management in dedicated stroke units. It is also likely that treatment decisions will be based more and more on an individual patient's cerebrovascular physiology rather than strict time limits. The approach will be to permanently open the occluded vessel with drugs and/or devices as rapidly as possible while protecting vulnerable cells with neuroprotective drugs or devices.

Secondary prevention of stroke

Once an ischemic stroke has occurred, the patient is at an increased risk for a second event, especially over the ensuing days or weeks.[30] The first step in secondary prevention is to determine the cause of the stroke, if possible. If there is a mechanical cause that can be corrected such as significant carotid stenosis or patent foramen ovale (PFO), then

---

Table 2.3 Basic management of patients with acute ischemic stroke[20]

- *Body position*: the patient should be supine in the bed.
- *Oxygen*: all stroke victims should initially be placed on supplemental oxygen.
- *Blood pressure*: both elevated and low blood pressure are associated with poor outcomes after stroke.[41] There are no definite guidelines for blood pressure levels immediately after AIS. Ischemic brain loses its autoregulation so the oxygen available for tissue becomes completely dependent on perfusion pressure which in turn is dependent on mean arterial blood pressure. Prior to reperfusion, blood pressure should remain high. Blood pressure no higher than 185/110 is the recommended level for administration of IV t-PA, and 180/105 for the initial 24 hours after IV t-PA treatment. After reperfusion, there is the risk of reperfusion injury (i.e., hemorrhage and edema), particularly at higher blood pressures. If pressures drop, particularly with worsening of clinical status, normotonic fluids without glucose should be used for resuscitation. Pressors can be considered in some cases, especially to encourage collateral blood flow in patients with defined proximal occlusive disease.
- *Hyperglycemia*: patients with elevated blood glucose following AIS have poorer outcomes.[42] In general, the desired blood glucose levels are 80–140 mg/dl.
- *Temperature*: fever should be treated to normothermia. Hypothermia is being tested to see if it improves outcomes from AIS.
- *Antithrombotic agents*: the standard timing of antithrombotic agents is 24 hours after the administration of IV t-PA or other reperfusion modalities. Patients who are not candidates for thrombolysis or other reperfusion treatments should be administered aspirin within 48 hours after onset of the stroke.

AIS, acute ischemic stroke; t-PA, tissue plasminogen activator.

procedures to correct the lesion should be considered in some cases. There are established data to support carotid endarterectomy over medical management in surgical candidates who have a >70% stenosis of the symptomatic carotid artery.[31] The benefits and risks of carotid stenting versus carotid endarterectomy are being evaluated in clinical trials.[32] Transcatheter devices and increasingly less-invasive open surgical approaches to close PFO are available, but have not yet been shown to be superior to medical management.[33,34] Vertebral and intracranial artery stenoses can be treated with angioplasty and stenting if the patient remains symptomatic on optimal medical treatment, and clinical trials will address the proper role of the use of stents in this setting.[35,36]

Table 2.4 Recommended goals for stroke risk factors[31,43]

Blood pressure	<120/70
Total cholesterol	<200
Low-density lipoprotein	<100 (in diabetics, <70)
Smoking cessation	
Maximum alcohol	2 drinks per day for males; 1 drink per day for females
Exercise 5 days per week	
Normal body weight	

Table 2.5 Options for antiplatelet therapy[31,40]

- Aspirin alone at doses of 81–325 mg daily has been shown to be effective in multiple trials
- Clopidogrel at 75 mg daily is effective (CAPRIE)[45]
- The combination of clopidogrel and Aspirin is not more effective than either agent alone, and the combination produces excess bleeding (CHARISMA[46], MATCH[47]).
- The combination of low dose aspirin and extended release dipyridamole is more effective than Aspirin alone (ESPS-2[48], ESPRIT[49]).
- The combination of low dose aspirin and extended release dipyridamole is as effective as clopidogrel in secondary stroke prevention (PRoFESS[50]).'

Identification of stroke risk factors is the next important step in secondary prevention. Hypertension, diabetes, smoking, and hyperlipidemia are the major risk factors, but obesity, inactivity, excess use of alcohol, and stress may also be important. *Table 2.4* summarizes recommended goals for risk factor management. The 'big three' of secondary stroke prevention are antithrombotic treatment, antihypertensive agents, and lipid-lowering treatment.[31] Recent randomized clinical trials have extensively addressed the importance of controlling these risk factors. Efforts to further drive down levels of blood pressure and low-density lipoprotein appear to be increasingly effective in stroke prevention.[37–39] Hypertension as a risk factor for stroke is discussed further in Chapter 3.

The last step in effective secondary prevention is selection of antithrombotic treatment.[40] In general, treatment with warfarin is the most effective way to prevent recurrent cardioembolic stroke. In most cases the International Normalized Ratio (INR) should be 2–3, with the exception of patients with artificial cardiac valves in which the INR should be 2.5–3.5. Warfarin is no better than aspirin in preventing recurrent stroke in patients with intracranial disease, and has a higher risk.[41] For all other types of strokes, including those caused by small vessel disease, antiplatelet treatment is recommended. *Table 2.5* summarizes the options for antiplatelet treatment and the trials supporting their use.

Case studies

Case study 1. Endovascular recanalization of a carotid T lesion

History

A 51-year-old woman with a history of hypertension and dyslipidemia presented on the morning of admission with right-sided hemiparesis. She was last seen well at 05:30, and subsequently found down by family member at 07:00.

Timeline

Emergency department
- 05:30–7:00, symptoms onset.
- 07:43, EMS dispatched.
- 08:10, Emergency Department arrival.
  - *Exam*: she could follow some commands, but was densely dysarthric with non-fluent aphasia, left gaze preference, right hemiparesis and neglect.
  - NIHSS score = 14 points.

- 08:30–8:40, head CT and CT angiography were obtained (**CS 1.1**):
  - a hyperdense left MCA sign was observed consistent with left M1 occlusion (A)
  - a normal left ICA bifurcation (B), but coronal intracranial images (C) show diminished flow in the distal left ICA as well as the M1 and A1 segments consistent with a carotid T occlusion
  - the CT perfusion study was incompletely processed, but a time-to-peak map suggests substantial left hemispheric ischemia (blue region) (D)
  - owing to the uncertainty of time from symptoms onset and the large clot located at the carotid T (likely to be unresponsive to IV t-PA alone), consent was obtained from the patient's husband for IA revascularization procedures.
- 09:10, anesthesia was started, with elective intubation.

Endovascular procedure

1 *Diagnostic angiography* (**CS 1.2**):
  - left ICA injection, posterior lateral views, shows mild cervical FMD (A,B), with a tortuous, redundant proximal cervical segment (A, arrows) as well as an acute intracranial occlusion (arrowheads), just above the level of the anterior choroidal artery
  - right ICA injection, anteroposterior (AP) projection, shows good cross-filling via the anterior communicating artery into the left A1 segments and distal ACA branches, with some leptomeningeal collateralization into the left MCA territory (arrows) (C).

2 *Interventional treatment* (**CS 1.2**, continued):
- 10:30, angiography during the procedure shows progressive reopening of the distal M1/proximal M2 occlusion, AP view (D).
  - A single pass of the Merci LX device resulted in excellent recanalization; the post-procedure AP (E) and a comparison of lateral views, pre-procedure (F, left) versus post-procedure (F, right).

3 *Pathology and post-treatment MRI scan* (**CS 1.3**):
  The procedure aspirated a <2-cm thrombus, shown attached to the Merci LX device (A), and alone (B). The pathologist's evaluation of the clot identified only fibrin and red blood cells.
- 12:16, transfer to Neuroscience ICU.
- 15:15, extubated.
- 16:45, brain MRI shows a small lesion on diffusion-weighted (arrowhead) (C) and FLAIR (D) sequences, with a normal intracranial MRA (E).

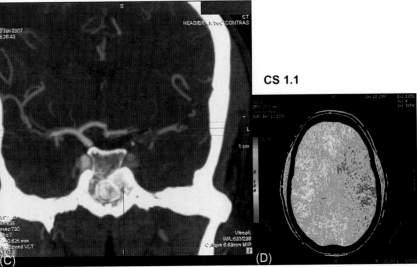

CS 1.1

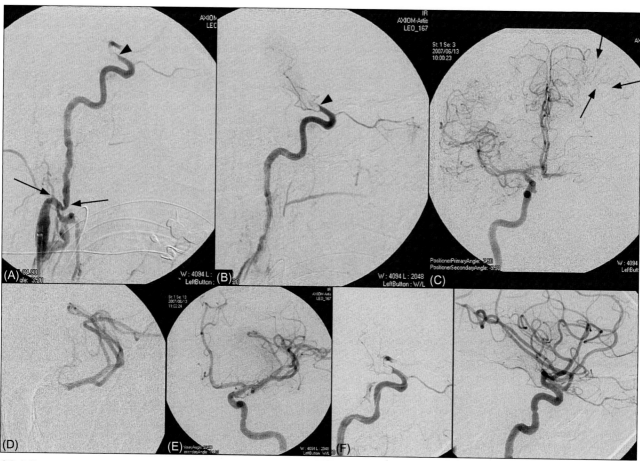

CS 1.2

Hospital course

- **Hospital day (HD) 2**, NIHSS score = 0 points.
- **HD3**, a TEE study showed a PFO with an interatrial septal aneurysm, and spontaneous right-to-left shunting. Anticoagulation was started.
- **HD4**, a lower-extremity venous Duplex ultrasound scan showed acute thrombus involving one posterior tibial vein and one peroneal vein in the left leg.
  - Laboratory studies were significant for elevated serum low-density lipoprotein, 116 mg/dl; and elevated C-reactive protein, 1.46 (normal range, 0–0.49 mg/dl).
- **HD5**, discharge to rehabilitation, on warfarin and statin treatment with no neurologic deficits.

Comments

This patient made an outstanding recovery from early endovascular recanalization. Her relatively low NIHSS score for a carotid T lesion probably reflected excellent native collateral circulation. The stroke etiology was likely paradoxical thromboembolism from a deep vein thrombosis, via a PFO. Secondary stroke prevention in this setting is controversial, with newer transcatheter and less invasive open surgical methods to close the PFO.[33,34] With identification of a deep vein thrombosis, warfarin for the first several months is an appropriate antithrombotic agent. Another risk factor to consider over the long-term is this patient's cervical FMD.

Case study 2. Intravenous thrombolysis with a 'matched' computed tomography perfusion study

History

A 75-year-old man with a history of tobacco use and hypertension presented to a local hospital with a left hemispheric stroke syndrome.

Timeline and hospital course

- 08:30, symptoms onset.
- 0 h 30 min, arrival at local hospital.
- 0 h 50 min, non-contrast head CT scan (not shown).
- 1 h, contact regional stroke center facility via 1-800 Stroke Hotline.

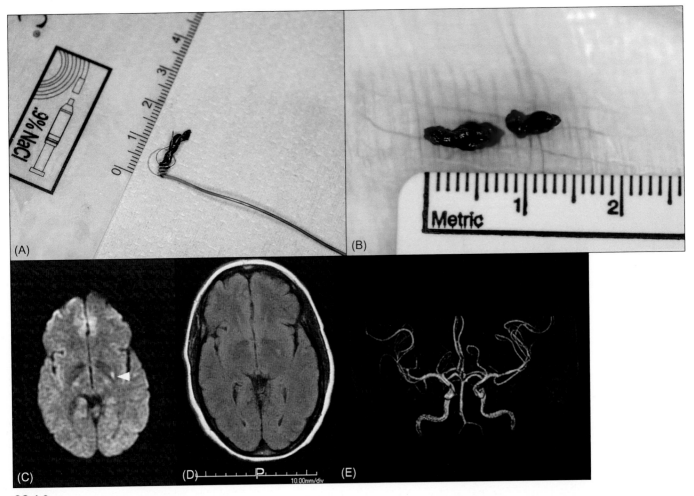

CS 1.3

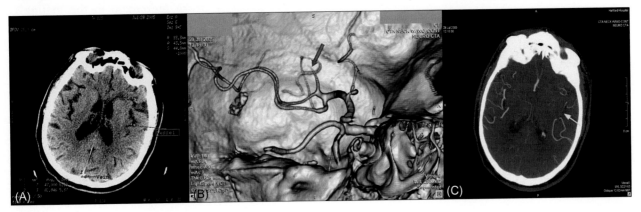

CS 2.1

- 2 h, bolus and infusion of IV t-PA started at local hospital.
- 3 h, arrival at regional stroke center:
  - initial NIHSS score = 22 points.
- 3 h 50 min, head CT scan (**CS 2.1**A):
  - CT angiography documents an M3 occlusion of the left MCA, shown on reconstructed three-dimensional study (B) (pink arrow) and maximum intensity projection (C) (yellow arrow).
- 4 h, CT perfusion (**CS 2.2**):
  - processing of the CT scan, and decision, with the neurointerventional team, to not pursue an endovascular procedure. The low-density lesion most prominent on the cerebral blood flow map (a black–dark blue region)

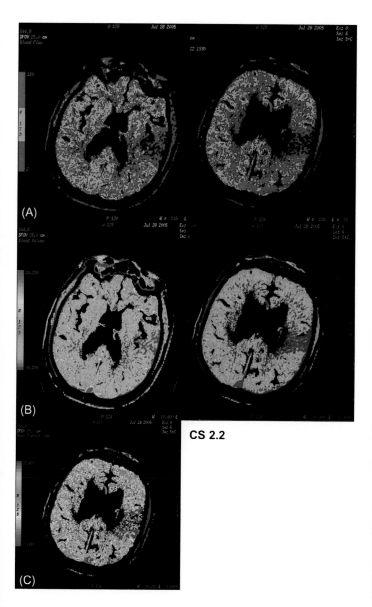

CS 2.2

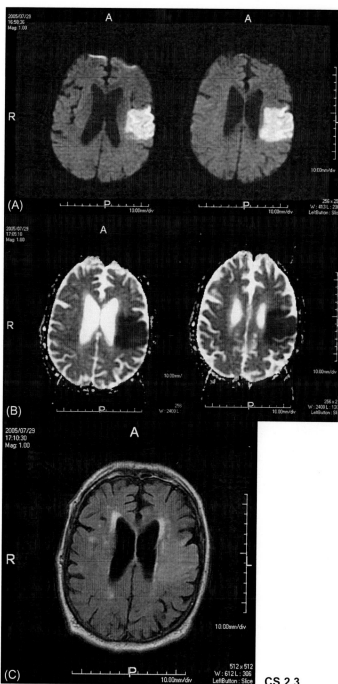

CS 2.3

(A) matches that on the cerebral blood volume (blue) (B) and mean transit time maps (blue) (C), indicating no viable penumbra (a 'matched' pattern).

- **HD2**
  - MRI (**CS 2.3**) on the next day, diffusion-weighted image sequences (A) and apparent diffusion coefficient map (B), corroborated the lesion on the previous day's CT perfusion scan as a wedged-shaped infarct. The final lesion on the FLAIR sequence (C) is comparable with the area of low cerebral blood volume (**CS 2.2**B).
- **HD6**
  - The patient is discharged to rehabilitation with a predominantly expressive aphasia, and some early return of right leg strength
  - Hospital discharge NIHSS score = 12 points.

Comments

The initial clinical evaluation upon arrival at the tertiary care center suggested a wide area of ischemia involving an occlusion in the first- or second-order left MCA. However, CT angiography showed a more peripheral third-order (M3) occlusion, and the largely matched cerebral blood flow and cerebral blood volume lesions suggested no ischemic penumbra at risk that would benefit from an endovascular procedure.[12,26,51,52]

Despite a relatively high initial NIHSS score (>20 points), the Stroke Team decided not to offer additional treatments beyond IV thrombolysis. The subsequent MRI scan confirmed a peripheral frontoparietal lesion. The patient's early recovery during the acute hospitalization was encouraging and validated this clinical decision.

Case study 3. Hemicraniectomy for the malignant middle cerebral artery syndrome

History and exam

A 56-year-old man was hospitalized for pneumonia. Two days later, he developed a right hemispheric stroke syndrome, with dysarthria, left hemiplegia, and hemineglect.

Timeline

HD1   Acute stroke symptoms onset.

HD3   Transfer to the regional stroke center.
Serial head CT scans (**CS 3.1**):

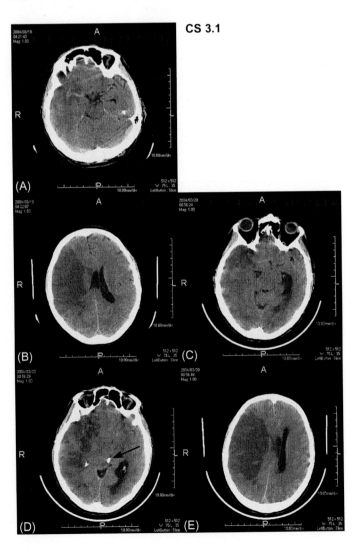

CS 3.1

HD4   Admission head CT scan shows an early large right MCA stroke (A,B).
- *Exam*: alert and conversant; left hemianopia and hemineglect; dense left hemiplegia. NIHSS score = 16 points.
- Neurosurgery consult to consider hemicraniectomy.

HD6   Deteriorating mental status prompted repeat head CT scan (C–E):
- Extensive right uncal herniation has markedly obscured the entire posterior fossa, with pressure on the midbrain and trapping of the contralateral left ventricle (C), midline shift of the calcified pineal gland (arrow) (D), and well-delineated MCA-territory infarct with subfalcine herniation (E).

HD6   **Hemicraniectomy (CS 3.2)**. The patient's wife was consented for this procedure.
- Following a large curvilinear incision from the anterior tragus back toward the occipital bone and to the midline of scalp (A, left), burr holes are made (A, right), and a wide skull bone window is removed (B).
- The exposed brain shows signs of elevated intracranial pressure, with engorged superficial veins (C). Following this craniotomy, the dura is closed with the addition of fascia latae from the scalp (arrows) (D).

HD7   **Postoperative day 1**, Neuroimaging (**CS 3.3**):
- head CT scan shows severe edema, pushing brain beyond the former skull margin, with some normalization toward midline. A single transaxial view (A) and composite views (B,C) demonstrate how the infarcted brain extends beyond the skull margin. A postoperative lateral skull film shows the stapled wound (D), and three-dimensional CT scan shows a postoperative AP view (E).

HD15   **Transfer to acute rehabilitation.**
Day 60 Recovery:
- Walking 80–100 feet, holding a quad cane in the right hand.
- Left shoulder subluxation on plain X-ray.

Day 84 Cranioplasty procedure (CS 3.4).
- The skull bone is replaced 3 months later (A): reconstructive surgery to encompass the region where the temporalis muscle was removed.
- Post-cranioplasty FLAIR MRI sequence (B,C). Note that there are small areas of apparently intact brain tissue within the large right MCA stroke.

(A)

(B)

(C)

(D)

- The patient following cranioplasty, with a widened palpebral fissure and mild lower facial paresis on the left (D).
- NIHSS score = 7 points, largely from residual left hemiparesis.

Day 104 Returns home from assisted living facility. Ambulating with quad cane.

A second patient, aged 51, underwent craniotomy for a malignant right MCA syndrome, and returned to the stroke clinic 1 year later, ambulatory, but with significant left hemiparesis (**CS 3.4**E). Note the left ankle–foot orthosis, and flexor posturing of the left hand.

CS 3.2

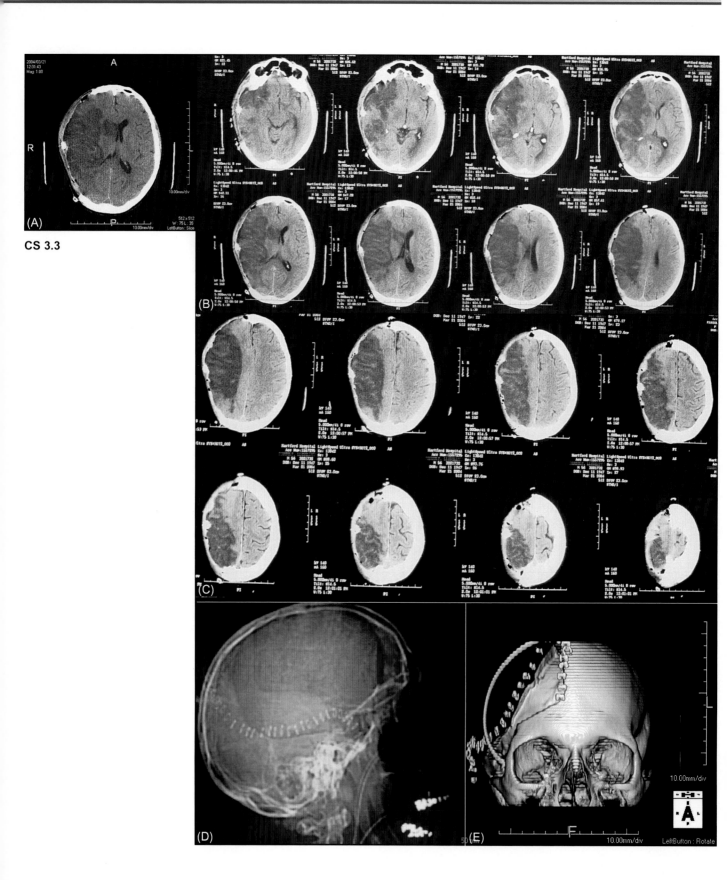

CS 3.3

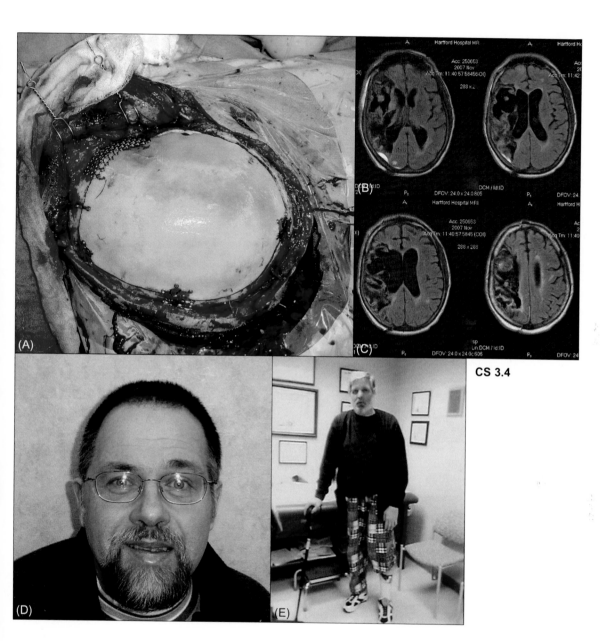

CS 3.4

Comments

Hemicraniectomy works. In an analysis of three randomized clinical trials, the procedure benefited not only survival but also short-term outcomes.[27] The time-to-randomization in this analysis was 45 hours, in order to begin the surgical procedure within 48 hours. Patient selection included an NIHSS score >15 points, with a diminished level of consciousness. The short-term survival was improved from 29% in the medical (placebo) arm, versus 78% in the treatment (surgical) arm. The number needed to treat to result in a single favorable outcome at 12 months, defined as modified Rankin Scale of ≤4 points, was two patients.

Key observations about these data are: (1) most case series and clinical trials work restrict the procedure to patients ≤60 years of age; (2) an excellent outcome from this life-threatening stroke may be defined by the ability to return to an ambulatory state, as the patients presented here did; and (3) the decision to intervene should be made within the first 12–48 hours, soon after acute treatments (e.g., IV t-PA and endovascular approaches) have been attempted yet before significant progression toward uncal herniation. In practice, hemicraniectomy is typically recommended for the treatment of non-dominant hemisphere strokes, but can also be considered for highly selected patients with left hemispheric stroke.

Some of the functional recovery seen with hemicraniectomy may relate to the salvaging of brain tissue within the ischemic penumbra (**CS 3.4**B,C). The patches of spared brain presumably avert pressure necrosis against the adjacent skull when that tissue acutely swells.

References

1. Warach S. Tissue viability thresholds in acute stroke: the 4-factor model. *Stroke* 2001; **32**: 2460–1.

2. Tilley B, Lyden P, Brott T, Lu M, Levine S, Welch K. Total quality improvement method for reduction of delays between emergency department admission and treatment of acute ischemic stroke. *Arch Neurol* 1997; **54**: 1466–74.

3. Alberts M, Hademenos G, Latchaw R, et al. Recommendations for the establishment of primary stroke centers. *JAMA* 2000; **283**: 3102–19.

4. Alberts M, Latchaw R, Selman W, et al. Recommendations for comprehensive stroke centers: a consensus statement from the Brain Attack Coalition. *Stroke* 2005; **36**: 1597–618.

5. Fisher M. Recommendations for advancing development of acute stroke therapies: Stroke Therapy Academic Industry Roundtable 3. *Stroke* 2003; **34**: 1539–46.

6. Brott T, Bogousslavsky J. Treatment of acute ischemic stroke. *N Engl J Med* 2000; **343**: 710–22.

7. del Zoppo G. Stroke and neurovascular protection. *N Engl J Med* 2006; **354**: 553–5.

8. National Institute of Neurological Disorders and Stroke rt-PA Stroke Study Group. Tissue plasminogen activator for acute ischemic stroke. *N Engl J Med* 1995; **333**: 1581–7.

9. Smith W, Sung G, Starkman S, et al., for the MERCI Trial Investigators. Safety and efficacy of mechanical embolectomy in acute ischemic stroke: results of the MERCI Trial. *Stroke* 2005; **36**: 1432–40.

10. McDougall C, Clark W, Mayer T, et al. The Penumbra Stroke Trial: safety and effectiveness of a new generation of mechanical devices for clot removal in acute ischemic stroke [abstract]. International Stroke Conference (New Orleans) 2008; LB4.

11. Konstas A-A, Choi J, Pile-Spellman J. Neuroprotection for ischemic stroke using hypothermia. *Neurocrit Care* 2006; **4**: 168–78.

12. Molina C, Saver J. Extending reperfusion therapy for acute ischemic stroke: emerging pharmacological, mechanical, and imaging strategies. *Stroke* 2005; **36**: 2311–20.

13. Saver J. Time is brain-quantified. *Stroke* 2006; **37**: 263–6.

14. Marler JR, Tilley BC, Lu M, et al. Early stroke treatment associated with better outcome: The NINDS rt-PA Stroke Study. *Neurology* 2000; **55**: 1649–55.

15. Hacke W, Donna G, Fieschi C, et al. Association of outcome with early stroke treatment: pooled analysis of ATLANTIS, ECASS, and NINDS rt-PA stroke trials. *Lancet* 2004; **363**: 768–74.

16. Hacke W, Kaste M, Bluhmki E, et al. Thrombolysis with alteplase 3 to 4.5 hours after acute ischemic stroke. *N Engl J Med* 2008; **359**: 1317–29.

17. Furlan A, Higashida R, Katzan I, Abou-Chebl A. Intra-arterial thrombolysis in acute ischemic stroke. In: Lyden P, ed. *Thrombolytic Therapy for Stroke*. Totowa, NJ: Humana Press; 2001: 175–95.

18. Furlan A, Higashida R, Wechsler L, et al. Intra-arterial prourokinase for acute ischemic stroke. The PROACT II Study: a randomized controlled trial. *JAMA* 1999; **282**: 2003–11.

19. Mattle H. Intravenous or intra-arterial thrombolysis? It's time to find the right approach for the right patient [editorial]. *Stroke* 2007; **38**: 2038–40.

20. Adams H, Jr, del Zoppo G, Alberts M, et al. Guidelines for the early management of adults with ischemic stroke: a guideline from the American Heart Association/ American Stroke Association Stroke Council, Clinical Cardiology Council, Cardiovascular Radiology and Intervention Council, and the Atherosclerotic Peripheral Vascular Disease and Quality of Care Outcomes in Research Interdisciplinary Working Groups. *Stroke* 2007; **38**: 1655–711.

21. Lindsberg P, Mattle H. Therapy of basilar artery occlusion: a systematic analysis comparing intra-arterial and intravenous thrombolysis. *Stroke* 2006; **37**: 922–8.

22. Agarwal P, Kumar S, Hariharan S, et al. Hyperdense middle cerebral artery sign: can it be used to select intra-arterial versus intravenous thrombolysis in acute ischemic stroke? *Cerebrovasc Dis* 2004; **17**: 182–90.

23. Zaidat O, Suarez J, Santillan C, et al. Response to intra-arterial and combined intravenous and intra-arterial thrombolytic therapy in patients with distal internal carotid artery occlusion. *Stroke* 2002; **33**: 1821–7.

24. Marder V, Chute D, Starkman S, et al. Analysis of thrombi retrieved from cerebral arteries of patients with acute ischemic stroke. *Stroke* 2006; **37**: 2086–93.

25. Rogalewski A, Schneider A, Ringelstein E, Schabitz W-R. Toward a multimodal neuroprotective treatment of stroke. *Stroke* 2006; **37**: 1129–36.

26. Kidwell CS, Alger JR, Saver JL. Beyond mismatch: evolving paradigms in imaging the ischemic penumbra with multimodal magnetic resonance imaging. *Stroke* 2003; **34**: 2729–35.

27. Stroke Unit Trialists Collaboration. How do stroke units improve patient outcomes? A collaborative systematic review of the randomized trials. *Stroke* 1997; **28**: 2139–44.

28. Schwab S, Steiner T, Aschoff A, *et al*. Early hemicraniectomy in patients with complete middle cerebral artery infarction. *Stroke* 1998; **29**: 1888–93.

29. Vahedi K, Hofmeijer J, Juettler E, *et al*. Early decompressive surgery in malignant infarction of the middle cerebral artery: a pooled analysis of three randomised controlled trials. *Lancet* 2007; **6**: 215–22.

30. Rothwell P, Warlow C. Timing of TIAs preceding stroke: time window for prevention is very short. *Neurology* 2005; **64**: 817–20.

31. Sacco R, Adams R, Albers G, *et al*. Guidelines for prevention of stroke in patients with ischemic stroke or transient ischemic attack. *Stroke* 2006; **37**: 577–617.

32. Furlan A. Carotid-artery stenting—case open or closed? [editorial]. *N Engl J Med* 2006; **355**: 1726–9.

33. Adams H, Jr. Cardiac disease and stroke: will history repeat itself? *Mayo Clin Proc* 2006; **81**: 597–601.

34. Kizer J, Devereux R. Patent foramen ovale in young adults with unexplained stroke. *N Engl J Med* 2005; **353**: 2361–72.

35. Fiorella D, Levy E, Turk A, *et al*. US multicenter experience with the Wingspan stent system for the treatment of intracranial atheromatous disease: periprocedural results. *Stroke* 2007; **38**: 881–7.

36. Zaidat O, Klucznik R, Chaloupka J, *et al*. An NIH-funded multicenter registry on the use of the Wingspan intracranial stent for high-risk patients with symptomatic intracranial arterial stenosis [abstract]. International Stroke Conference (San Francisco) 2007; LB3.

37. PROGRESS Group. Randomised trial of a perindopril-based blood-pressure-lowering regimen among 6105 individuals with previous stroke or transient ischaemic attack. *Lancet* 2001; **358**: 1033–41.

38. Schrader J, Lüders S, Kulschewski A, *et al.*; MOSES Study Group. Morbidity and Mortality After Stroke, Eprosartan Compared with Nitrendipine for Secondary Prevention: principal results of a prospective randomized controlled study (MOSES). *Stroke* 2005; **36**: 1218–26.

39. The Stroke Prevention by Aggressive Reduction in Cholesterol Levels (SPARCL) Investigators. High-dose atorvastatin after stroke or transient ischemic attack. *N Engl J Med* 2006; **355**: 549–59.

40. Albers G, Amarenco P, Easton J, Sacco R, Teal P. Antithrombotic and thrombolytic therapy for ischemic stroke: The Seventh ACCP Conference on Antithrombotic and Thrombolytic Therapy. *Chest* 2004; **3**: S483–512.

41. Chimowitz MI, Lynn MJ, Howlett-Smith H, *et al*. Comparison of warfarin and aspirin for symptomatic intracranial arterial stenosis. *N Engl J Med* 2005; **352**(13): 1305–16.

42. Castillo J, Leira R, Garcia M, Serena J, Blanco M, Davalos A. Blood pressure decrease during the acute phase of ischemic stroke is associated with brain injury and poor stroke outcome. *Stroke* 2004; **35**: 520–6.

43. Baird T, Parsons M, Phanh T, *et al*. Persistent poststroke hyperglycemia is independently associated with infarct expansion and worse clinical outcome. *Stroke* 2003; **34**: 2208–14.

44. Chobanian A, Bakris G, Black H, *et al*. Seventh report of the Joint National Committee on prevention, detection, evaluation, and treatment of high blood pressure (JNC 7 – Complete Version). *Hypertension* 2003; **42**: 1206–52.

45. CAPRIE Steering Committee. A randomised, blinded, trial of clopidogrel versus aspirin in patients at risk of ischaemic events (CAPRIE). *Lancet* 1996; **348**: 1329–39.

46. Bhatt D, Fox K, Hacke W, *et al*. Clopidogrel and aspirin versus aspirin alone for the prevention of atherothrombotic events. *N Engl J Med* 2006; **354**: 1706–17.

47. Diener H-C, Bogousslavsky J, Brass L, *et al*. Aspirin and clopidogrel compared with clopidogrel alone after recent ischaemic stroke or transient ischaemic attack in high-risk patients (MATCH): randomised, double-blind, placebo-controlled trial. *Lancet* 2004; **364**: 331–7.

48. Diener H, Cunha L, Forbes C, Sivenius J, Smets P, Lowenthal A. European Stroke Prevention Study 2. Dipyridamole and acetylsalicylic acid in the secondary prevention of stroke. *J Neurol Sci* 1996; **143**: 1–13.

49. The ESPRIT Study Group. Aspirin plus dipyridamole versus aspirin alone after cerebral ischaemia of arterial origin (ESPRIT): randomised controlled trial. *Lancet* 2006; **367**: 1655–73.

50. Sacco R, Diener H-C, Yusuf S, *et al.* Aspirin and extended-release dipyridamole versus clopidogrel for recurrent stroke. *N Engl J Med* 2008; **359**: 1238–51.

51. Lev M, Segal A, Farkas J, *et al.* Utility of perfusion-weighted CT imaging in acute middle cerebral artery stroke treated with intra-arterial thrombolysis: Prediction of final infarct volume and clinical outcome. *Stroke* 2001; **32**: 2021–8.

52. Wintermark M, Reichhart, Thiran JP, *et al.* Prognostic accuracy of cerebral blood flow measurement by perfusion computed tomography, at the time of emergency room admission in acute stroke patients. *Ann Neurol* 2002; **51**: 417–32.

Further reading

Adams H, Jr, del Zoppo G, Alberts M, *et al.* Guidelines for the early management of adults with ischemic stroke: a guideline from the American Heart Association/ American Stroke Association Stroke Council, Clinical Cardiology Council, Cardiovascular Radiology and Intervention Council, and the Atherosclerotic Peripheral Vascular Disease and Quality of Care Outcomes in Research Interdisciplinary Working Groups. *Stroke* 2007; **38**: 1655–711.

del Zoppo G. Stroke and neurovascular protection. *N Engl J Med* 2006; **354**: 553–5.

Lyden P. *Thrombolytic Therapy for Stroke*. Totowa, NJ: Humana Press; 2001. This textbook provides a superb overview of the development of IV and IA thrombolysis for AIS, along with case studies.

Sacco RL, Adams R, Albers G, *et al.* Guidelines for prevention of stroke in patients with ischemic stroke or transient ischemic attack. *Stroke* 2006; **36**: 577–617.

Warach S. Tissue viability thresholds in acute stroke: The 4-factor model. *Stroke* 2001; **32**: 2460–1.

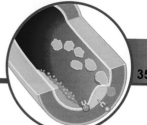
Hypertension as a Risk Factor for Stroke

Introduction

Studies of stroke etiology and hypertension treatment provide overwhelming evidence for a log-linear and continuous causative association between hypertension and stroke.[1, 2] It is now well-established that, after age, hypertension is the most significant risk factor for both ischemic and hemorrhagic stroke (3.1).[2, 3] The treatment of hypertension is highly effective in the primary prevention of stroke and the reduction of stroke incidence and mortality.[4, 5]

The Perindopril Protection Against Recurrent Stroke (PROGRESS) and Morbidity and Mortality After Stroke: Eprosartan compared with Nitrendipine for Secondary Prevention (MOSES) studies showed that blood pressure (BP) lowering also reduces the risk of secondary strokes and other major vascular events in patients who have had a previous transient ischemic attack (TIA) or stroke.[6, 7] This chapter will focus on the role of the angiotensin receptor blockers (ARBs) in the prevention of ischemic stroke in patients with hypertension.

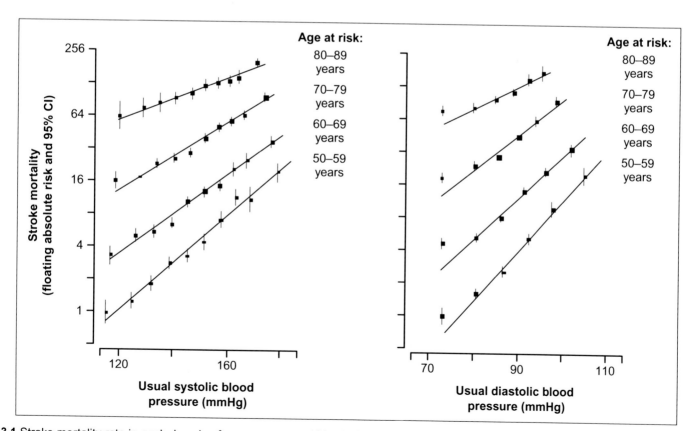

3.1 Stroke mortality rate in each decade of age versus usual blood pressure at the start of that decade.[3] CI, confidence interval.

Hypertension and increased stroke risk

Arterial hypertension arises from a combination of increased cardiac output and increased peripheral resistance. In adults, hypertension is defined as a consistent measurement of systolic blood pressure (SBP) of 140 mmHg or higher, and/or a diastolic blood pressure (DBP) of 90 mmHg or higher. Around 74.5 million people in the United States aged 20 and over have high blood pressure; less than half have it well-controlled (U.S. Centers for Disease Control and Prevention). Elevated SBP is an independent risk factor for stroke,[8] but stroke risk approximately doubles with each 7.5 mmHg increase in the level of DBP.[1]

In contrast to secondary hypertension, which is associated with underlying disorders such as kidney disease, the pathophysiology of essential hypertension is not fully understood. Accounting for over 90% of cases of hypertension, it appears to be influenced by multiple factors, including genetic mutations, and inadequate environmental factors, including high dietary salt intake and factors facilitating overweight and obesity. Many mechanisms are implicated in the development of essential hypertension, including endothelial dysfunction, vascular overreactivity to vasoconstrictors, increased sympathetic nervous system activity, disrupted renal salt regulation, and disturbances in the renin-angiotensin-aldosterone (RAAS) regulatory system (**3.2**).[9]

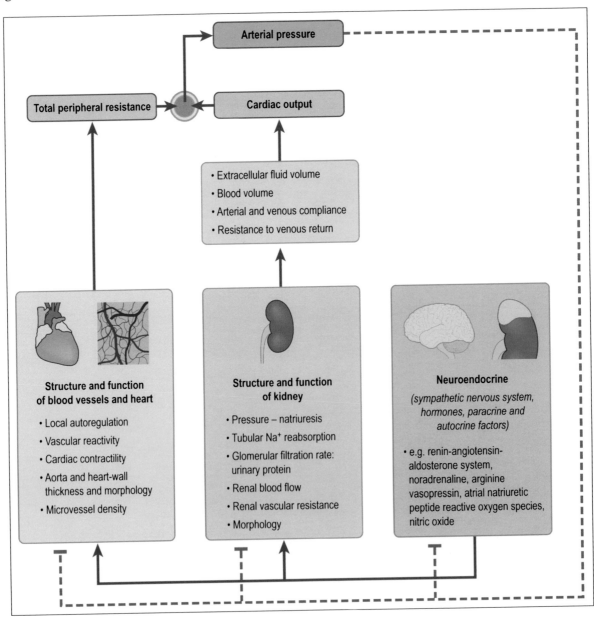

3.2 Mechanisms of arterial blood pressure regulation.[10]

Chronic essential hypertension is complex, and there is variation between individuals as to the pathophysiology involved in its genesis. However, whether as a cause or consequence of the hypertensive state, several aspects contribute to the elevation of ischemic and hemorrhagic stroke risk. Intracerebral vascular changes are the main reason why hypertension is a leading risk factor for stroke.[11] Abnormal vascular endothelial responses are observed in hypertensive patients, whose vessels show enhanced sensitivity to the vasoconstrictor endothelin-1 and reduced levels of vasodilators such as nitric oxide (NO) (3.3). Endothelial damage resulting from increased intraluminal pressure can increase interactions between leukocytes and endothelial cells, leading to local thrombus formation and eventual fibrinoid necrosis (3.3).[12]

Hypertension also increases the extent and severity of atheroma by accelerating the arteriosclerotic process, with increased low-density lipoprotein (LDL) oxidation and foam cell formation occurring in hypertensive vessels. Plaques form initially in the large extracerebral carotid artery, and progressively spread to the circle of Willis and the smaller intracerebral arteries.[13] Recent research has demonstrated that, even in prehypertensive patients, elevated BP is associated with a thickening of the carotid intima-media and, by inference, an increased risk of ischemic stroke.[14] As demonstrated in the VALUE study, early intervention with antihypertensives is essential in reducing the risk of stroke.[15] The currently recommended classes of antihypertensives are summarized in *Box 3.1*. Their benefits in terms of stroke prevention largely accrue through their BP lowering properties, such that factors relating to patient tolerance and interactions with pre-existing conditions or medications are often used to guide treatment choice.[16] However, some drugs may confer additional benefits distinct from antihypertensive effects alone; this is discussed further below.

The risk of hemorrhage from the small cerebral arteries is also increased in hypertension, largely due to progressive hypertrophy of the muscular vessel wall and the endothelium. These adaptive structural changes in the resistance vessels reduce the vessel wall tension, but cause increased peripheral vascular resistance that may compromise the collateral circulation and enhance the risk for ischemic events, particularly distal to a stenosis. Hypertension is often observed in conjunction with other cardiovascular risk factors for stroke, for instance, atrial fibrillation[17] or bilateral carotid stenosis.[18]

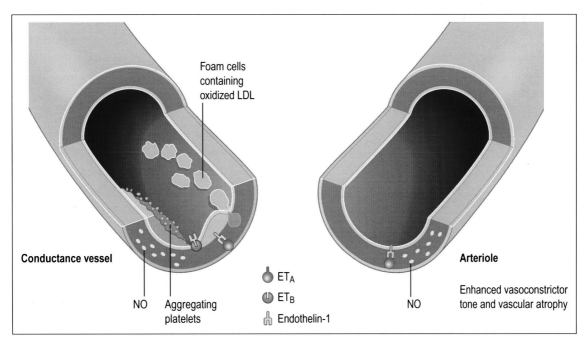

3.3 Decreased activity of NO and enhanced type A endothelin receptor (ETA)-mediated vasoconstrictor activity of endothelin-1 in the hypertensive vasculature result in increased vascular tone and medial hypertrophy, which increase systemic vascular resistance. The imbalance in endothelial factor activity leads to a proatherosclerotic state conducive to the oxidation of low-density lipoprotein (LDL), the adhesion and migration of monocytes, and the formation of foam cells. These activities ultimately lead to the development of atherosclerotic plaques.[9]

The renin-angiotensin-aldosterone system and regulation of blood pressure

Abnormal activity of the RAAS is implicated in cardiovascular, cerebrovascular and renovascular disease. The RAAS is a complex regulatory system that influences BP through multiple actions on the vascular endothelia, kidneys and sympathetic nervous system (**3.4**). Renin is released by the juxtaglomerular cells in the kidneys, and catalyses the conversion of angiotensinogen, which is secreted into the circulation from the liver, into angiotensin I, an oligopeptide hormone (**3.4**). Angiotensin-converting enzyme 1 (ACE1) converts angiotensin I into angiotensin II. Angiotensin II modulates vascular tone, renal function, aldosterone and vasopressin release, and sympathetic nervous system effects, through binding to the angiotensin II receptor type 1 (AT_1).[19] This specific, high-affinity receptor for angiotensin II is expressed in the adrenal zona glomerulosa, vascular smooth muscle, heart, kidney, liver, brain, and anterior pituitary gland. ACE1 is expressed throughout the body, but high concentrations are found in the lungs.

Angiotensin stimulates the secretion of aldosterone from the adrenal cortex; this causes increased renal reabsorption of sodium and water. Further mechanisms for increasing BP are the ACE-mediated degradation of circulating vasodilatory bradykinins, and the angiotensin II-induced release of antidiuretic hormone (ADH; vasopressin) from the posterior pituitary gland. Crosstalk between the RAAS and the sympathetic nervous system also occurs to a considerable extent.[20] Angiotensin II effects norepinephrine release from sympathetic nerve terminals via stimulation of presynaptic angiotensinergic receptors, and amplifies alpha receptor-mediated vasoconstrictor responses to norepinephrine, increasing BP further. Angiotensin II has also been shown to inhibit baroreceptor control of heart rate.

In hypertension, aberrant activation and/or regulation of the RAAS leads to prolonged elevation of BP through prolonged activity of ACE and increased levels of angiotensin II. Angiotensin II increases BP through several mechanisms.[21] Following binding to AT_1 in vascular endothelia, angiotensin II stimulates contraction in vascular smooth muscle cells via a Gq protein-coupled inositol trisphosphate (IP_3)-dependent mechanism. In the kidneys, angiotensin II has complex effects on renal circulation and glomerular filtration rate, restricting blood flow through constriction of the glomerular arterioles, but also causing vasodilatory prostaglandin release. Angiotensin II also acts on the adrenal cortex, causing it to release aldosterone, which causes the kidneys to retain sodium and lose potassium. Increased sodium levels then lead to increased BP; consequently, a high salt diet is a risk factor for hypertension and can also cause dysfunction of the RAAS.[22] Aldosterone also has systemic effects,[23] and synergy between the actions of aldosterone and angiotensin II has been observed, both in the central and peripheral circulation.[24] In addition to vascular endothelial effects, angiotensin II can cause prothrombic aggregation of platelets and production of plasminogen activator inhibitor (PAI)-1 and PAI-2.[25]

Renal and cardiovascular effects are also mediated by the more recently discovered ACE2 pathway,

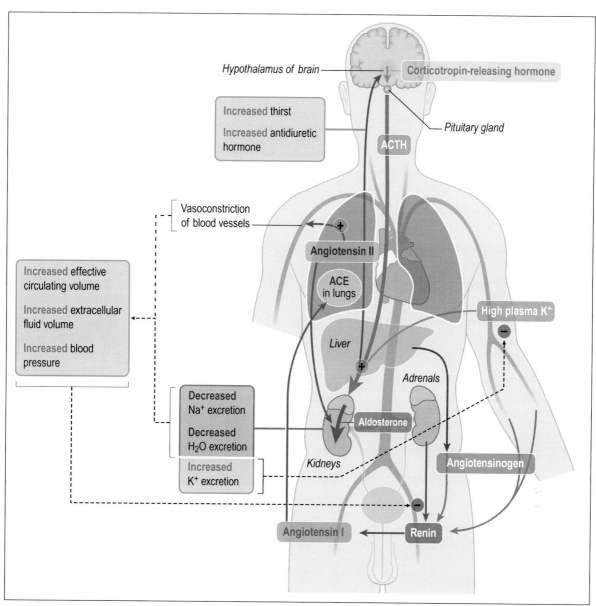

3.4 The renin-angiotensin system.[23]

which converts angiotensin I to angiotensin (1–9) and angiotensin II to angiotensin (1–7). The ACE2/angiotensin (1–7) receptor axis is thought to inhibit fibrosis, inflammation, thrombosis and cell proliferation, and to modulate renin-angiotensin system (RAS) activity, with significant pathophysiological implications in clinical conditions such as hypertension, myocardial ischemia and heart failure.[26]

Further angiotensin II receptors, types 2, 3 and 4, are expressed in the vascular endothelia and other tissues. Unlike AT_1, they are not solely involved in regulation of BP; AT_2, for instance, is highly expressed during fetal development

and may modulate growth pathways. In addition to their effects on BP and hemodynamics, recent studies have provided evidence that angiotensin receptors influence a range of other processes, including tumorigenesis, cardiomyopathy, autoimmune disease and even longevity.[27]

Angiotensin II receptor blockers as antihypertensives

Pharmaceutical blockade of the RAAS has been shown to be beneficial in patients with hypertension, stroke, acute myocardial infarction, chronic systolic heart failure, and diabetic renal disease.[28] Currently, two classes of drugs are used to target the RAAS: ACE inhibitors and ARBs. ACE inhibitors reduce the rate of conversion of angiotensin I to angiotensin II, ameliorating its hypertensive effects. ARBs target the AT_1 receptor, preventing its activation by angiotensin II. This causes vasodilation as opposed to vasoconstriction, reduces vasopressin and aldosterone secretion, and diminishes the induction of norepinephrine by angiotensin II.

Since the introduction of losartan in 1995, seven commercially available ARBs have been developed, which differ slightly in their structure and properties (*Table 3.1*). The ARBs are small (~0.4 kDa) molecules containing a tetrazole ring and one or more imidazole rings. Key clinical features include pressor inhibition, or the amount of blockade of the BP-raising effect of angiotensin II, at trough plasma levels. However, overall antihypertensive efficacy is dependent on a number of other factors, including AT_1 receptor affinity, bioavailability, and biological half-life.

ARBs in clinical use

The pathophysiology of hypertension is complex and varies considerably between individuals. For this reason, many patients fail to respond to one or more drugs, or may experience unpleasant side effects. Physicians frequently need to try several drugs before finding one that allows the patient to achieve control of their hypertension with minimal adverse effects. Combination therapies are increasingly being used, and are being tested in ongoing trials.[29] ARBs are frequently used in patients who do not tolerate ACE inhibitors as trials have shown them to have side-effect profiles comparable to placebos.[30] For instance, side effects such as cough or angioedema experienced by patients intolerant to ACE inhibitors occur less frequently upon switching to ARBs (this is thought to be because ARBs do not affect bradykinin breakdown). The most frequently used antihypertensives are ACE inhibitors, beta-blockers, calcium channel blockers (CCBs), and diuretics. In terms of efficacy and safety, several large-scale studies have established the first-line

Table 3.1 Characteristics of the seven prescribed angiotensin II receptor blockers

ARB	Marketed as	Pressor inhibition (trough) (%)	Biological half-life, (hours)	Renal/ hepatic clearance (%)	Daily dosage (mg)
Losartan	Cozaar (Merck), generic 2010	25–40	2	10/90	50–100
Candesartan	Blopress, Atacand, Amias, Ratacand (AstraZeneca/ Takeda)	50	9	60/40	4–32
Eprosartan	Teveten (Abbott)	30	20	30/70	400–800
Valsartan	Diovan (Novartis)	30	6	30/70	80–320
Irbesartan	Aprovel, Karvea, Avapro (Sanofi-Aventis/Bristol Myers-Squibb)	60	11–15	1/99	150–300
Telmisartan	Micardis (Boehringer Ingelheim), Targit (Pfizer India Ltd)	40	24	1/99	40–80
Olmesartan	Benicar, Olmetec (Daiichi-Sankyo)	60–74	14–16	40/60	10–40

therapy using ARBs as a worthwhile option for hypertension; however, current European Society of Hypertension (ESH) and European Society of Cardiology (ESC) guidelines state that first-line treatment choice should be made on an individual basis, according to patient need, since there are few differences in terms of BP lowering between the classes of medication available.[31]

ARBs are indicated in patients with essential hypertension, and especially in diabetic hypertensive patients to prevent any vascular and/or renal complications. There are few contraindications for ARBs, but they are not used in pregnancy or in patients with bilateral renal artery stenosis. Such patients may experience renal failure with ARBs, due to blockade of the efferent arteriole AT_1 receptors causing an abrupt fall in glomerular filtration rate.

ARBs are well tolerated by most individuals. The most common side effects are low BP, dizziness, headache, hyperkalemia and drowsiness. Less frequently, diarrhea, muscle cramps, pharyngitis and rash can occur. More serious, but rare, side effects are kidney failure, liver failure, allergic reactions, a decrease in white blood cells, and angioedema.

ARBs and cardiovascular risk
Overall, BP lowering by ARBs results in reduced cardiovascular risk in patients with hypertension versus no treatment at all. Although data from the VALUE study published in 2004 prompted doubts over the relative efficacies of ARBs versus other antihypertensives in the prevention of myocardial infarction (MI) and cardiovascular death,[15, 32] this is thought to be a result of confounding factors created by the design of the VALUE trial itself. Subsequently, a post hoc direct comparison in the subgroup of patients who received monotherapy throughout with either comparator drug demonstrated that, when the data were corrected for changes in BP from baseline, which were not equal as was anticipated in the original study design, rates of MI prevention were comparable.[33] Furthermore, the VALUE study showed both the rate of new-onset diabetes and the incidence rate for heart failure to be lower in valsartan-treated patients.[15] More recently, the NAVIGATOR study demonstrated that the use of valsartan for 5 years, versus placebo and alongside lifestyle modification, led to a relative reduction of 14% in the incidence of diabetes in patients with impaired glucose tolerance and cardiovascular risk factors.[34] The rate of cardiovascular events was not significantly reduced, but did not increase in the patients receiving valsartan. Recent data from the MOSES study, comparing

the ARB eprosartan with the CCB nitrendipine indicated no significant differences in MI risk among cardiovascular secondary endpoints.[7] Definitive evidence from prospective trials and further meta-analyses of large-scale comparisons of ARBs with other antihypertensives will be needed to clarify their impact on cardiovascular risk independent of their BP-lowering capacity.

ARBs and stroke prevention
As antihypertensives, ARBs reduce stroke risk by countering the damaging effects of prolonged elevated blood pressure. In promoting the widening of arteries and acting as anti-fibrotics, they also reduce the likelihood of thrombus formation. There is also evidence for BP-independent effects on stroke risk, from comparative trials with other antihypertensives.

Comparing the stroke outcomes of the most significant trials of five ARBs, some show greater risk reduction compared to other therapies, others less (*Table 3.2*). There remain questions over whether ARBs consistently offer enhanced primary or secondary stroke protection in all patients. Trial design and choice of comparator regimens are challenging in studies of antihypertensives, as few patients remain on study drug monotherapy, and subjects may have a range of comorbidities.

Losartan
The Losartan Intervention for Endpoint reduction in hypertension (LIFE) study compared losartan to atenolol in 9000 patients, and demonstrated 40% stroke risk reduction with the ARB in patients with systolic hypertension. Although overall BP differences were small, losartan was better at lowering SBP in diabetic patients. However, only 10% of patients were on losartan or atenolol monotherapy by the end of the LIFE study; combination treatments with ACE inhibitors and/or CCBs were required to control hypertension in the majority of subjects. This was the first study to demonstrate the BP-independent impact of ARBs on primary stroke risk.[35]

Telmisartan and valsartan
Studies of telmisartan in stroke prevention have been less conclusive, with no additional benefit seen in comparisons to ACE inhibitors or, for secondary prevention, placebo.[36] In contrast, valsartan compared favorably to non-ARB regimens in the large-scale Kyoto Heart Study, involving over 3000 high-risk Japanese patients with uncontrolled hypertension.[37]

Table 3.2 Stroke risk reduction data from head-to-head RCT comparisons of ARBs and other hypertensives

ARB	Study	No. patients	Key stroke data
Losartan	LIFE	9000	Significant stroke reduction vs atenolol (25%; $P = 0.001$), with significant reductions in a subset without clinical vascular disease (34%; $P < 0.001$) and in ischemic (27%; $P = 0.001$), atherothrombotic (27%; $P = 0.002$), and fatal (35%; $P = 0.032$) stroke in a subanalysis of specific subtypes
			Secondary prevention: significant reduction ($n = 26$ vs $n = 46$; $P = 0.017$) in subtype focused analysis
Telmisartan	PRoFESS	20 332	Secondary prevention: no significant recurrent stroke reduction (primary endpoint) vs placebo when initiated within 90 days after ischemic stroke
	TRANSCEND	5926	Overall stroke: no significant stroke reduction vs placebo in ACE inhibitor-intolerant patients with cardiovascular disease or diabetes/end-organ damage
	ONTARGET	25 620	Demonstrated non-inferiority to the ACE inhibitor ramipril for primary prevention of vascular events in a high-risk population
Eprosartan	MOSES	1352	Secondary prevention: significant reduction vs nitrendipine (25%; $P = 0.026$) in fatal/nonfatal cerebrovascular events
Candesartan	SCOPE	4937	Significant reduction vs placebo (28%; $P = 0.04$) in nonfatal stroke in elderly hypertensive patients, with significant all-stroke reduction in a subset with isolated systolic hypertension
	E-COST	2048	Primary prevention: no significant stroke reduction vs conventional antihypertensive treatment, with a 29% increased risk with candesartan in patients without history of stroke or MI
			Secondary prevention: significant stroke reduction for candesartan vs conventional antihypertensive treatment in patients with past stroke or MI (61%; $P < 0.01$)
Valsartan	Kyoto Heart Study	3031	Significant reduction vs non-ARB regimens (45%; $P = 0.015$) in stroke or transient ischemic attack in Japanese patients with hypertension at high risk for cardiovascular events

Candesartan

Candesartan reduced primary and secondary stroke risk compared with atenolol in the Study on Cognition and Prognosis in the Elderly (SCOPE) trial,[38] but showed no primary preventive effect in E-COST, although some secondary protective benefit was seen in patients with prior MI or stroke.[39]

Eprosartan

Eprosartan performed well against the CCB, nitrendipine, in the MOSES study of secondary stroke prevention, further detailed below. Additionally, in a 6-week study in patients with hypertension, eprosartan 600 mg once daily was more effective than the beta-blocker atenolol 50 mg once daily in reducing central SBP, but atenolol was associated with a greater effect on aortic stiffness.[40]

A meta-analysis by the Blood Pressure Lowering Treatment Trialists' Collaboration (BPLTTC) compared a range of trials of different treatment regimens. The results showed clear benefits of BP-lowering treatment regardless of starting BP, but did not show a significant difference in the effect of regimen on cardiovascular events or overall BP lowering.[41] However, the analysis covered only the short-term to medium-term effects of the regimens studied; differences may arise between the effects of different regimens in each baseline BP group in the longer term.

Additional benefits of ARBs

In addition to their efficacy as antihypertensives, ARBs may have been shown to confer additional benefits not demonstrated for ACE inhibitors. However, since the evidence base comprises just a small number of studies, all of the following claims are not confirmed and the use of ARBs cannot be recommended in the specified conditions. Data from randomized controlled trails (RCTs) and meta-analyses have shown that in addition to stroke prevention, ARBs can improve renal function, ameliorate atherosclerosis and atrial fibrillation, and potentially reduce risk in left ventricular dysfunction.[42] For example, significant reduction of left ventricular hypertrophy (LVH) was observed with irbesartan but not with atenolol in the SILVHIA study, despite comparable efficacy in terms of BP lowering.[43] Other ARBs have also been shown to produce regression of LVH. With regard to atrial fibrillation, key data from the LIFE study demonstrated a 33% reduction in new-onset atrial fibrillation with losartan compared to atenolol.[35] Irbesartan was also shown to reduce atrial fibrillation risk by 65% when combined with amiodarone, versus amiodarone alone.[44] Conversely, there is little evidence to suggest that ARBs offer any greater protection from MI than ACE inhibitors.

A significant negative association between ARBs and Alzheimer's disease was first reported in 2008. A retrospective analysis of five million patient records found that different types of commonly used antihypertensive medications had very different outcomes. Patients taking ARBs were 35–40% less likely to develop Alzheimer's disease than those using other antihypertensives.[45] However, despite initially promising findings in the ONTARGET trial, further analysis has shown rates of cognitive decline and dementia are unaffected by BP lowering in patients taking antihypertensives over several years, regardless of the treatment used.[46]

Secondary stroke prevention using eprosartan

While the efficacy of ARBs in primary prevention of stroke is established, their use for secondary prevention in patients who have already experienced a stroke or TIA has only recently been explored. Intensive lowering of BP with an ACE inhibitor and diuretic has shown promise in reducing secondary risk.[47] The MOSES trial asked whether a similar effect would be seen with an ARB, eprosartan, in comparison to nitrendipine. Nitrendipine showed significant reductions in stroke versus placebo in the Syst-Eur trial in elderly patients.[48] As an ARB, eprosartan works by blocking binding of angiotensin II to AT_1 receptors, with subsequent effects on renal and vascular function. Direct pressor inhibition is 100% at peak concentrations, declining to around 30% over 24 hours. Eprosartan also results in inhibition of sympathetic norepinephrine production. The MOSES study group hypothesized that ARBs may have greater cerebroprotective effects due to selective blocking of AT_1 receptors but not AT_2 receptors, although this is not proven. Therefore, in hypertensive stroke patients, for the same level of BP control, it was hypothesized that eprosartan would be more effective than nitrendipine in reducing cerebrovascular and cardiovascular morbidity and mortality. The rationale for choosing these drugs was the cerebroprotective experimental effects of various sartans, and the positive results of the Syst-Eur study in which nitrendipine reduced primary stroke and dementia. The primary endpoint was the composite of all-cause mortality and the number of cardiovascular and cerebrovascular events, including all recurrent events.

The MOSES multicenter RCT recruited 1352 patients aged under 85, of whom 681 received eprosartan 600 mg daily, and 671 were given 10 mg daily nitrendipine (a CCB). All patients had hypertension and had experienced a stroke, TIA or intracranial hemorrhage within the two years preceding enrollment. Exclusion criteria included carotid artery stenosis of >70%, atrial fibrillation requiring anticoagulants, or unstable angina.

Over a mean follow-up of 2.5 years, BP reduction was observed to be similar in both groups, with no differences in adverse events between the two. With regard to the primary endpoint (all-cause mortality and cardiovascular and cerebrovascular events), a higher event incidence was observed in the nitrendipine group in comparison to the eprosartan one ($P = 0.014$).[7] By the end of the trial, monotherapy with eprosartan was received by 234 patients (34.4%); monotherapy with nitrendipine was given to 222

(33.1%). A similar reduction in BP was observed in both groups, over the same time course and to a comparable extent, without any significant differences during the study period. At the final visit, the mean office BP was 137.5/80.8 mmHg with eprosartan-based regimens and 136.0/80.2 mmHg with nitrendipine-based regimens. Across the entire study population receiving antihypertensive treatment, 236 further cerebrovascular events occurred, 102 in the eprosartan group and 134 in the nitrendipine group (IDR 0.75, 95% CI 0.58–0.97; *Table 3.3*). This equates to a 25% reduction in risk with eprosartan ($P = 0.026$).

Table 3.3 MOSES study: cerebrovascular events

Event	Eprosartan (*n* = 681)	Nitrendipine (*n* = 671)
Stroke	31	39
TIA	66	92
Intracranial hemorrhage	5	3
Total	**102**	**134**

In the high-risk patients recruited by the MOSES trial, a protective effect independent of BP lowering was demonstrated through the lower frequency of first cardiovascular events when using eprosartan compared to nitrendipine. MOSES was the first study comparing an ARB with a CCB for secondary stroke prevention; further trials with different agents are planned. Including TIA as an endpoint in such trials is subject to debate, as diagnostic confirmation can be variable. MOSES is similar to LIFE in the sense that it is the first trial to show a reduction in stroke risk in patients with comparable BP control to a comparator drug, in this case in secondary prevention.

Conclusion

Hypertension is a major risk factor for stroke, and arises via a number of mechanisms. The RAAS has significant influence on renal, vascular and nervous BP regulatory systems, modulated via the binding of angiotensin II to its receptor. Targeting the RAAS with ACE inhibitors or ARBs is a safe

and effective means of reducing BP. ARBs perform well in comparative trials in terms of stroke risk reduction. There is considerable evidence for additional cardiovascular and renoprotective benefits with ARBs, and eprosartan was also shown to act as a secondary stroke preventer in the MOSES study. Further studies are needed to establish the role of the ARBs in secondary prevention, in subsets of patients, in combination with other classes of drug, and in new treatment modalities. The latter includes the use of ARBs in acute stroke, currently under investigation in Scandinavian Candesartan Acute Stroke Trial (SCAST) using candesartan, following suggested beneficial effects in the ACCESS trial.[49]

References

1. MacMahon S, Peto R, Cutler J, *et al*. Blood pressure, stroke, and coronary heart disease. Part 1, Prolonged differences in blood pressure: prospective observational studies corrected for the regression dilution bias. *Lancet* 1990; **335**: 765–74.
2. Shimizu Y, Kato H, Lin CH, Kodama K, Peterson AV, Prentice RL. Relationship between longitudinal changes in blood pressure and stroke incidence. *Stroke* 1984; **15**: 839–46.
3. Lewington S, Clarke R, Qizilbash N, Peto R, Collins R; Prospective Studies Collaboration. Age-specific relevance of usual blood pressure to vascular mortality: a meta-analysis of individual data for one million adults in 61 prospective studies. *Lancet* 2002; **360**: 1903–13.
4. Collins R, Peto R, MacMahon S, *et al*. Blood pressure, stroke, and coronary heart disease. Part 2, Short-term reductions in blood pressure: overview of randomised drug trials in their epidemiological context. *Lancet* 1990; **335**: 827–38.
5. MRC trial of treatment of mild hypertension: principal results. Medical Research Council Working Party. *Br Med J (Clin Res Ed)* 1985; **291**: 97–104.
6. Randomised trial of a perindopril-based blood-pressure-lowering regimen among 6,105 individuals with previous stroke or transient ischaemic attack. *Lancet* 2001; **358**: 1033–41.
7. Schrader J, Lüders S, Kulschewski A, *et al*; MOSES Study Group. Morbidity and Mortality After Stroke, Eprosartan Compared with Nitrendipine for Secondary Prevention: principal results of a prospective randomized controlled study (MOSES). *Stroke* 2005; **36**: 1218–26.

8. Kannel WB, Wolf PA, McGee DL, Dawber TR, McNamara P, Castelli WP. Systolic blood pressure, arterial rigidity, and risk of stroke. The Framingham study. *JAMA* 1981; **245**: 1225–9.

9. Oparil S, Zaman MA, Calhoun DA. Pathogenesis of hypertension. *Ann Intern Med* 2003; **139**: 761–76.

10. Cowley AW, Jr. The genetic dissection of essential hypertension. *Nat Rev Genet* 2006; 7: 829–40.

11. Johansson BB. Vascular mechanisms in hypertensive cerebrovascular disease. *J Cardiovasc Pharmacol* 1992; **19** (Suppl 3): S11–15.

12. Fredriksson K, Nordborg C, Kalimo H, Olsson Y, Johansson BB. Cerebral microangiopathy in stroke-prone spontaneously hypertensive rats. An immunohistochemical and ultrastructural study. *Acta Neuropathol* 1988; **75**: 241–52.

13. Johansson BB. Hypertension mechanisms causing stroke. *Clin Exp Pharmacol Physiol* 1999; **26**: 563–5.

14. Manios E, Michas F, Tsivgoulis G, *et al*. Impact of prehypertension on carotid artery intima-media thickening: actual or masked? *Atherosclerosis* 2011; **214**: 215–9.

15. Julius S, Kjeldsen SE, Weber M, *et al*. Outcomes in hypertensive patients at high cardiovascular risk treated with regimens based on valsartan or amlodipine: the VALUE randomised trial. *Lancet* 2004; **363**: 2021–31.

16. Mancia G, De Backer G, Dominiczak A, *et al*; ESH-ESC Task Force on the Management of Arterial Hypertension. 2007 ESH-ESC Practice Guidelines for the Management of Arterial Hypertension: ESH-ESC Task Force on the Management of Arterial Hypertension. *J Hypertens* 2007; **25**: 1751–62.

17. Verdecchia P, Reboldi G, Gattobigio R, *et al*. Atrial fibrillation in hypertension: predictors and outcome. *Hypertension* 2003; **41**: 218–23.

18. Rothwell PM, Howard SC, Spence JD. Relationship between blood pressure and stroke risk in patients with symptomatic carotid occlusive disease. *Stroke* 2003; **34**: 2583–90.

19. Catt KJ, Mendelsohn FA, Millan MA, Aguilera G. The role of angiotensin II receptors in vascular regulation. *J Cardiovasc Pharmacol* 1984; **6** (Suppl 4): S575–86.

20. Grassi G. Renin-angiotensin-sympathetic crosstalks in hypertension: reappraising the relevance of peripheral interactions. *J Hypertens* 2001; **19**: 1713–6.

21. Hall JE (ed). *Guyton and Hall Textbook of Medical Physiology*, 12th edn. Philadelphia: Saunders; 2010.

22. Drenjančević-Perić I, Jelaković B, Lombard JH, Kunert MP, Kibel A, Gros M. High-salt diet and hypertension: focus on the renin-angiotensin system. *Kidney Blood Press Res* 2011; **34**: 1–11.

23. Briet M, Schiffrin EL. Aldosterone: effects on the kidney and cardiovascular system. *Nat Rev Nephrol* 2010; **6**: 261–73.

24. Xue B, Beltz TG, Yu Y, *et al*. Central interactions of aldosterone and angiotensin II in aldosterone- and angiotensin II-induced hypertension. *Am J Physiol Heart Circ Physiol* 2011; **300**: H555–64.

25. Skurk T, Lee Y-M, Hauner H. Angiotensin II and its metabolites stimulate PAI-1 protein release from human adipocytes in primary culture. *Hypertension* 2001; **37**: 1336–40.

26. Castro-Chaves P, Cerqueira R, Pintalhao M, Leite-Moreira AF. New pathways of the renin–angiotensin system: the role of ACE2 in cardiovascular pathophysiology and therapy. *Expert Opin Ther Targets* 2010; **14**: 485–96.

27. Stegbauer J, Coffman TM. New insights into angiotensin receptor actions: from blood pressure to aging. *Current Opin Nephrol Hypertens* 2011; **20**: 84–8.

28. Ma TK, Kam KK, Yan BP, Lam YY. Renin–angiotensin-aldosterone system blockade for cardiovascular diseases: current status. *Br J Pharmacol* 2010; **160**: 1273–92.

29. Werner C, Pöss J, Böhm M. Optimal antagonism of the renin-angiotensin-aldosterone system: do we need dual or triple therapy? *Drugs* 2010; **70**: 1215–30.

30. Farsang C, Fisher J. Optimizing antihypertensive therapy by angiotensin receptor blockers. In: Fischer J, Ganellin CR (eds). *Analogue-Based Drug Discovery*. Weinheim: Wiley-VCH; 2006: 157–67.

31. Mancia G, De Backer G, Dominiczak A, *et al*; Management of Arterial Hypertension of the European Society of Hypertension; European Society of Cardiology. 2007 Guidelines for the Management of Arterial Hypertension: The Task Force for the Management of Arterial Hypertension of the European Society of Hypertension (ESH) and of the European Society of Cardiology (ESC). *J Hypertens* 2007; **25**: 1105–87.

32. Strauss MH, Hall AS. Angiotensin receptor blockers may increase risk of myocardial infarction: unraveling the ARB-MI paradox. *Circulation* 2006; **114**: 838–54.

33. Julius S, Weber MA, Kjeldsen SE, *et al*. The Valsartan Antihypertensive Long-Term Use Evaluation (VALUE)

Trial: outcomes in patients receiving monotherapy. *Hypertension* 2006; **48**: 385–91.

34. Navigator Study Group, McMurray JJ, Holman RR, *et al.* Effect of valsartan on the incidence of diabetes and cardiovascular events. *N Engl J Med* 2010; **362**: 1477–90.

35. Wachtell K, Lehto M, Gerdts E, *et al.* Angiotensin II receptor blockade reduces new-onset atrial fibrillation and subsequent stroke compared to atenolol: The Losartan Intervention For End point reduction in hypertension (LIFE) study. *J Am College Cardiol* 2005; **45**: 712–19.

36. Yusuf S, Diener HC, Sacco RL, *et al.* Telmisartan to prevent recurrent stroke and cardiovascular events. *N Engl J Med* 2008; **359**: 1225–37.

37. Sawada T, Yamada H, Dahlöf B, Matsubara H; KYOTO HEART Study Group. Effects of valsartan on morbidity and mortality in uncontrolled hypertensive patients with high cardiovascular risks: KYOTO HEART Study. *Eur Heart J* 2009; **30**: 2461–9.

38. Papademetriou V, Farsang C, Elmfeldt D, *et al*; Study on Cognition and Prognosis in the Elderly study group. Stroke prevention with the angiotensin II type 1-receptor blocker candesartan in elderly patients with isolated systolic hypertension: The Study on Cognition and Prognosis in the Elderly (SCOPE). *J Am Coll Cardiol* 2004; **44**: 1175–80.

39. Suzuki H, Kanno Y; Efficacy of Candesartan on Outcome in Saitama Trial (E-COST) Group. Effects of candesartan on cardiovascular outcomes in Japanese hypertensive patients. *Hypertens Res* 2005; **28**: 307–14.

40. Dhakam Z, McEniery CM, Yasmin, Cockcroft JR, Brown MJ, Wilkinson IB, *et al.* Atenolol and eprosartan: differential effects on central blood pressure and aortic pulse wave velocity. *Am J Hypertens* 2006; **19**: 214–19.

41. Czernichow S, Zanchetti A, Turnbull F, *et al*; Blood Pressure Lowering Treatment Trialists' Collaboration. The effects of blood pressure reduction and of different blood pressure-lowering regimens on major cardiovascular events according to baseline blood pressure: meta-analysis of randomized trials. *J Hypertens* 2011; **29**: 4–16.

42. Siragy HM. Comparing angiotensin II receptor blockers on benefits beyond blood pressure. *Adv Ther* 2010; **27**: 257–84.

43. Malmqvist K, Ohman KP, Lind L, Nyström F, Kahan T. Long-term effects of irbesartan and atenolol on the renin-angiotensin-aldosterone system in human primary hypertension: the Swedish Irbesartan Left Ventricular Hypertrophy Investigation versus Atenolol (SILVHIA). *J Cardiovasc Pharmacol* 2003; **42**: 719–26.

44. Madrid AH, Bueno MG, Rebollo JM, *et al.* Use of irbesartan to maintain sinus rhythm in patients with long-lasting persistent atrial fibrillation: a prospective and randomized study. *Circulation* 2002; **106**: 331–6.

45. Li NC, Lee A, Whitmer RA, *et al.* Use of angiotensin receptor blockers and risk of dementia in a predominantly male population: prospective cohort analysis. *BMJ* 2010; **340**: b5465. doi: 10.1136/bmj.b5465.

46. Anderson C, Teo K, Gao P, *et al*; ONTARGET and TRANSCEND Investigators. Renin-angiotensin system blockade and cognitive function in patients at high risk of cardiovascular disease: analysis of data from the ONTARGET and TRANSCEND studies. *Lancet Neurol* 2011; **10**: 43–53.

47. PROGRESS Collaborative Group. Randomised trial of a perindopril-based blood-pressure-lowering regimen among 6,105 individuals with previous stroke or transient ischaemic attack. *Lancet* 2001; **358**: 1033–41.

48. Staessen JA, Fagard R, Thijs L, *et al.* Randomised double-blind comparison of placebo and active treatment for older patients with isolated systolic hypertension. The Systolic Hypertension in Europe (Syst-Eur) Trial Investigators. *Lancet* 1997; **350**: 757–64.

49. Sandset EC, Murray G, Boysen G, *et al*; SCAST Study Group. Angiotensin receptor blockade in acute stroke. The Scandinavian Candesartan Acute Stroke Trial: rationale, methods and design of a multicentre, randomised- and placebo-controlled clinical trial (NCT00120003). *Int J Stroke* 2010; **5**: 423–7.

INDEX